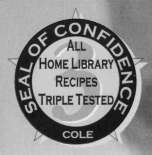

# babies and toddlers

# good food

*from the Home Library Test Kitchen*

**Cole's Home Library Cookbooks**
**Glen Ellen, California**

# babies and toddlers

## CONTENTS

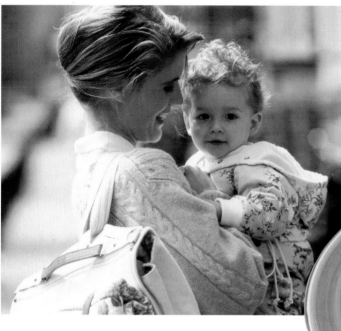

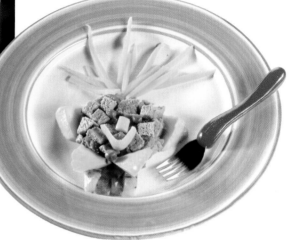

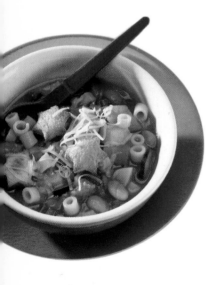

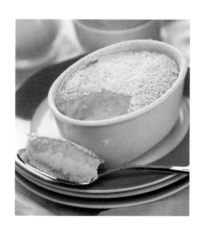

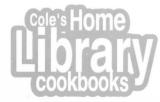

Cole's **Home Library cookbooks**

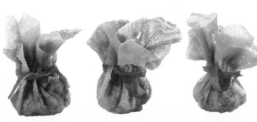

# good food

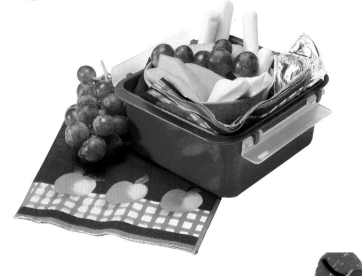

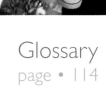

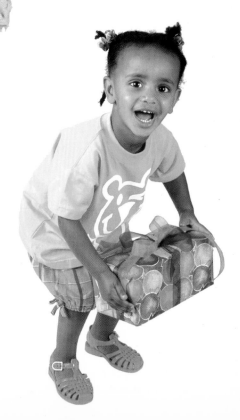

# learning about food for infants

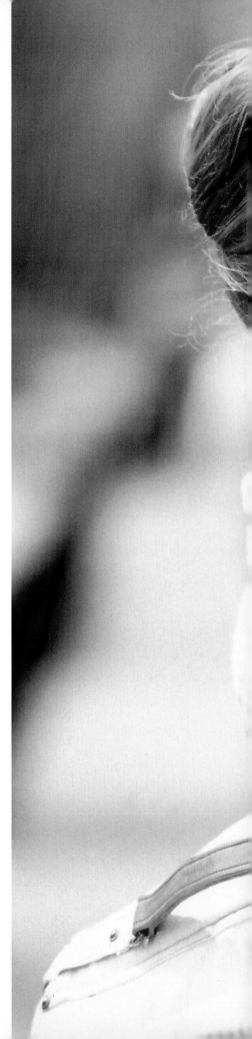

Let's be honest — food and eating are not only a vitally important part of living, they are also one of life's great pleasures. Having spent your whole life eating, and developing your own tastes and nutritional standards, it is now time to begin to pass your accrued wisdom onto the latest addition to your family. And while this might seem like a solemn task (and in the days to come, possibly a rather thankless one at times), there is no doubt that with a little common sense and a large dose of humor, you will find it not only manageable but also very rewarding as you watch your baby learn about food and the wonderfully sociable process of eating.

When you are poring over pyramid charts of the five food groups and agonizing over baby's lack of interest in your latest culinary offering, it is very easy to lose sight of the fact that learning about food can, and should, be fun.

The important thing is to use this book as a reference, and not as a set of rules that must be slavishly obeyed. Babies are individuals. They do things at different rates and early on can display very definite likes and dislikes. For every baby who eats cottage cheese with undisguised relish, there will be another (yours) who spits it in your eye every time. You can take it personally, or you can serve something else.

The trick is to remain flexible, be guided by your baby and, above all, try not to worry too much. Learning about food is an extended process and the least sensible approach is to feel guilty because *your* little bundle of joy appears to have been born with a cynical disregard for the five food groups. Go with the flow — your reward, in the short term, will be a baby who is soon eating family meals with you happily and, in the long term, the establishment of good eating habits for a lifetime.

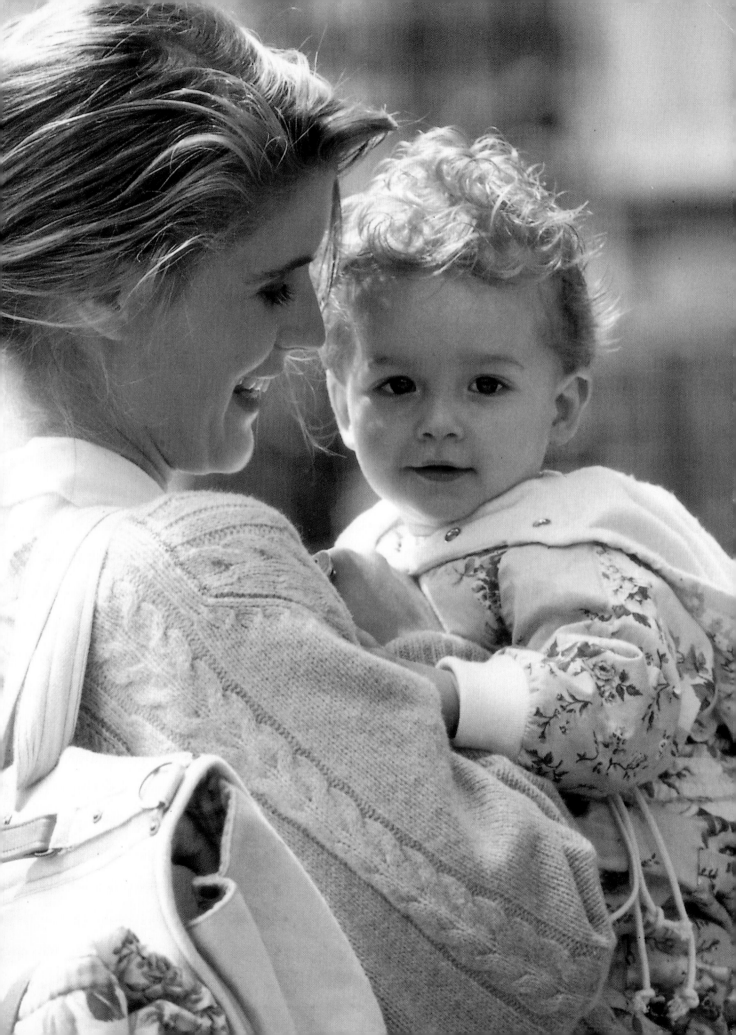

# Moms need feeding too!

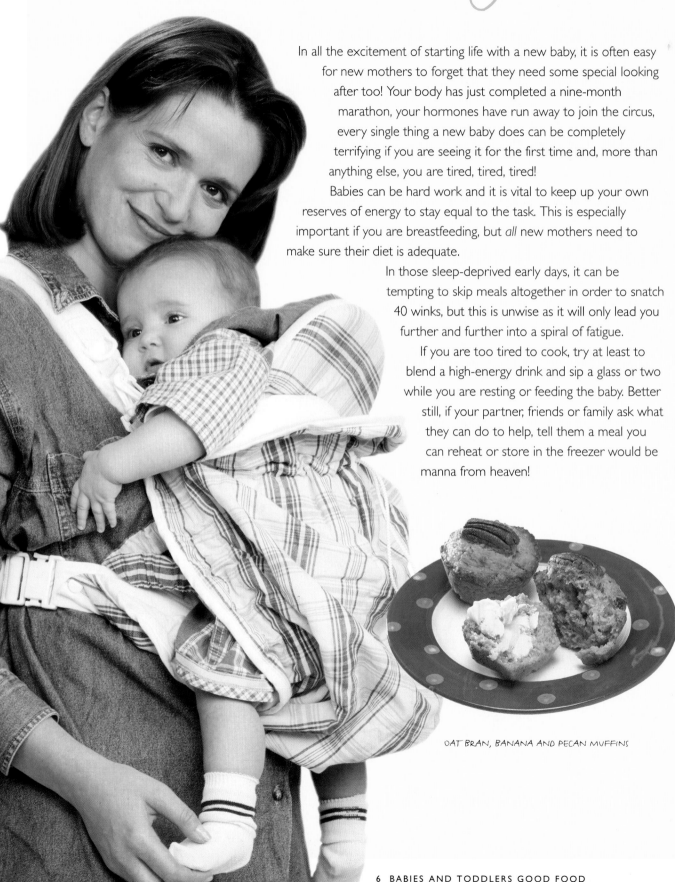

In all the excitement of starting life with a new baby, it is often easy for new mothers to forget that they need some special looking after too! Your body has just completed a nine-month marathon, your hormones have run away to join the circus, every single thing a new baby does can be completely terrifying if you are seeing it for the first time and, more than anything else, you are tired, tired, tired!

Babies can be hard work and it is vital to keep up your own reserves of energy to stay equal to the task. This is especially important if you are breastfeeding, but *all* new mothers need to make sure their diet is adequate.

In those sleep-deprived early days, it can be tempting to skip meals altogether in order to snatch 40 winks, but this is unwise as it will only lead you further and further into a spiral of fatigue.

If you are too tired to cook, try at least to blend a high-energy drink and sip a glass or two while you are resting or feeding the baby. Better still, if your partner, friends or family ask what they can do to help, tell them a meal you can reheat or store in the freezer would be manna from heaven!

OAT BRAN, BANANA AND PECAN MUFFINS

## oat bran, banana and pecan muffins

*You will need about 2 large overripe bananas for this recipe.*

**3/4 cup wholewheat
    self-rising flour**
**1 cup white
    self-rising flour**
**1/2 teaspoon apple-pie spice**
**1/2 cup oat bran**
**3 tablespoons brown sugar**
**1/2 cup pecans,
    chopped coarsely**
**1 cup mashed banana**
**1/4 cup vegetable oil**
**2 eggs, beaten lightly**
**1/3 cup skim milk**
**3 tablespoons golden syrup**
**12 pecans, extra**

Grease a 12-cup (1/3-cup-capacity) muffin pan.

Sift flours and spice into large bowl; stir in bran, sugar and chopped pecans. Add banana, then combined oil, eggs, milk and syrup; stir just until combined. Divide mixture among muffin tin cups; top with extra pecans. Bake at 400°F 20 minutes; turn onto wire rack to cool.

MAKES 12

*Best made on day of serving*

## tuna and ricotta potatoes

**4 large potatoes**
**6 oz can tuna in oil,
    drained, flaked**
**1 cup ricotta cheese**
**4 green onions, chopped finely**
**4 teaspoons baby capers**
**2 teaspoons finely grated
    lemon rind**
**6 tablespoons finely
    chopped parsley**
**2 cloves garlic, crushed**

Scrub potatoes well; pierce skin all over. Bake potatoes at 350°F about 1 1/2 hours or until tender. When cool enough to handle, cut 1/2 inch off top of each potato; scoop out and reserve flesh, leaving 1/4-inch shell. Combine potato flesh with remaining ingredients in medium bowl; divide mixture between potato shells. Place potatoes on baking sheet; bake, uncovered, about 15 minutes or until hot. Serve with yogurt, if desired.

MAKES 4

*Best made just before serving*

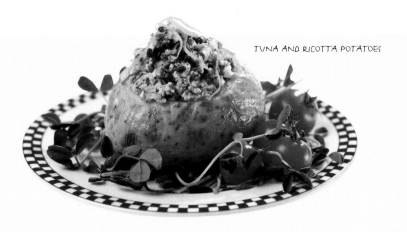

TUNA AND RICOTTA POTATOES

## fruit cup crush

**1 large mango,
    chopped coarsely**
**1 cup coarsely chopped
    watermelon**
**1/4 medium pineapple,
    chopped coarsely**
**1 1/2 tablespoons sugar**
**1 cup orange juice**

Blend or process fruit and sugar until smooth; add juice, blend until combined.

MAKES 4 CUPS

*Best made just before serving*

## banana smoothie

**1 medium banana,
    chopped coarsely**
**3/4 cup milk**
**1 1/2 tablespoons yogurt**
**3 tablespoons honey**
**1 scoop vanilla
    ice cream**
**4 ice cubes**

Blend or process all ingredients until smooth.

MAKES 2 CUPS

*Best made just before serving*

## mixed berry shake

**1 cup strawberries**
**1/2 cup raspberries**
**1/2 cup blueberries**
**1 1/2 tablespoons
    honey-flavored yogurt**
**2 teaspoons sugar**
**3/4 cup milk**
**1 scoop vanilla ice cream**

Blend or process all berries until pureed; strain through fine sieve into mixing bowl. Blend or process berry puree with remaining ingredients until smooth.

MAKES 2 CUPS

*Best made just before serving*

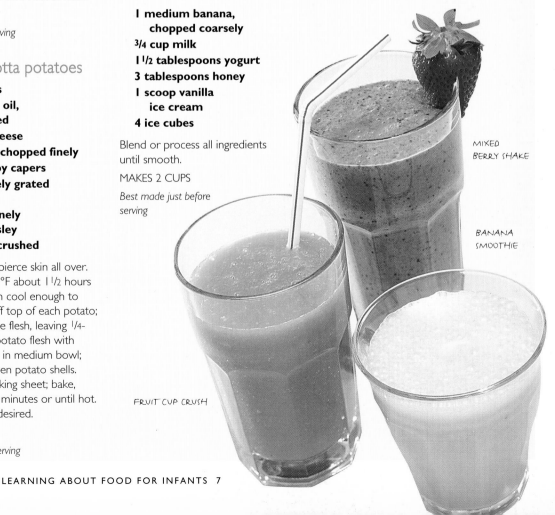

MIXED BERRY SHAKE

BANANA SMOOTHIE

FRUIT CUP CRUSH

# 0 to 4 months
## OFF TO A GOOD START

### Mother's milk

Breast milk is what nature designed for new babies. It contains exactly what they need in terms of nutrients, comes in perfect germ-free containers, and is always on hand at precisely the right temperature. Given these impeccable advantages, it would have to be the natural choice for a baby's first nutrition, wherever possible.

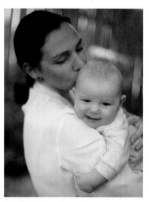

However, sometimes breastfeeding is just not an option, and if you are bottle-feeding your baby, you should take comfort from the knowledge that today's infant formulas are the nearest thing that science can get to breast milk. And of course, whether you choose breast or bottle, almost as important as nutrition in these early weeks is the wonderful intimacy that develops between you and your baby as feeding patterns are established. Everyone tells you about feeding, burping, colic and

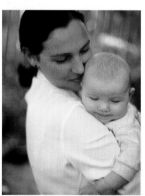

diaper rash. Nobody has ever come close to describing adequately that exquisite moment of communication when your gaze is held firmly by this extraordinary little stranger before the eyelids begin to droop with utter satisfaction.

But occasionally, it can be somewhat bewildering as well — some babies feed at regular intervals, others seem to want to graze non-stop around the clock, much to the alarm of their poor, sleep-starved mothers! Whether you are breastfeeding or bottle-feeding, your physician, local midwife or other early childhood health professional is an invaluable source of help and information for these early days. You will also meet other new mothers whose own experiences are reassuringly similar to yours.

### Thinking about weaning

Milk — your own, or an infant formula — is all the food a baby requires for the first four to six months of life. Deciding when to begin weaning baby onto solid food will depend on your own particular circumstances and should always be a gradual process to give you both time to adjust to the change.

After the simplicity of feeding your baby only milk for as long as six months, the idea of introducing solid food can seem a little daunting, especially as everyone you talk to is suddenly an expert on what to do and how to do it. A well-meaning relative will tell you that a big baby like yours needs solids to make him sleep through the night. Your neighbor will swear that cereals stopped her baby's reflux vomiting, and a woman at the checkout will point out your baby's chewed fists as evidence of excessive hunger. Do not get confused — none of these situations calls for weaning. Be guided by your baby and professional advice, and proceed at your own pace. After all, most people seem to have managed to learn to eat, even those whose mothers had begun to think it might never happen!

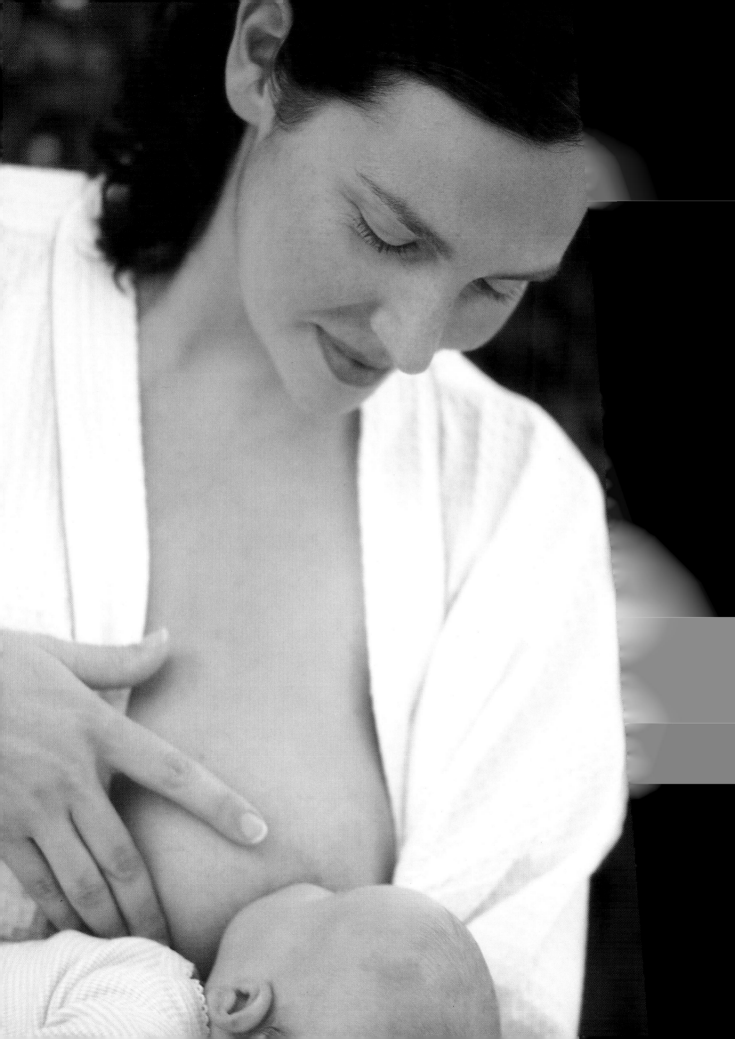

## First things first

So suddenly we are talking about food instead of just milk – a whole new ball game! There is no need to take a second mortgage for special new equipment, however. Whatever glossy catalogs might suggest to the contrary; baby's needs are really still very simple. To start, you will need small spoons without sharp edges – plastic are ideal – an unbreakable bowl and a supply of bibs – the one thing you can count on is a mess! Depending on the age of your baby, you will also need a high chair or something else for baby to sit in which is easy to wipe down.

Older toddlers can have their own little chair and table, unless you prefer them to sit on a booster seat at the main table. In either case, it is important to establish a specific location for eating – do not let your toddler walk and eat; make him sit and recognize a meal time and place.

## Cooking equipment

Food processors and hand-held blenders are great assets when preparing food for young babies who tend to like their purees absolutely smooth. However, a potato masher, ricer or food mill will also puree soft foods just as well and are less expensive. You can also push

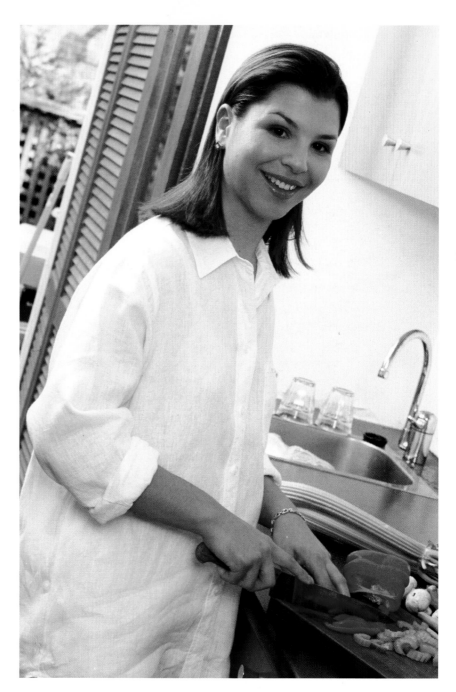

small amounts of soft food through a sieve to eliminate lumps.

## Kitchen hygiene

• Make sure you always have clean hands before starting to prepare any food.
• All feeding equipment and cooking utensils should be scrupulously clean, but, unlike bottles and nipples, there is no need to sterilize them.

• Use different clean chopping boards for raw meat and cooked foods, for poultry and vegetables, to avoid the risk of contamination.
• When preparing dry cereal, make only as much as required for each meal and discard any leftovers.
• NEVER save any uneaten portion of food from the feeding bowl – baby's saliva will have contaminated the remaining food. Discard it.

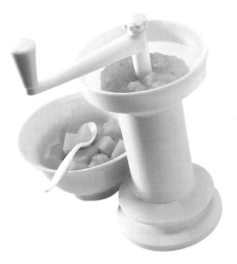

## Freezing

• Freeze single portions of food in ice cube trays or simply by dropping serving-sized spoonfuls onto a clean tray. Cover tightly and freeze. Once they are frozen, work quickly to place individual servings in freezer bags. Seal, label, date and return to the freezer.

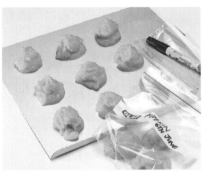

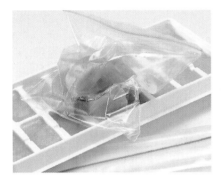

• Do not prepare vast amounts of food – you will never get through it. Ensure that food is rotated so oldest food is used first.
• Remove only the exact number of cubes required for each meal.
• Always thaw frozen portions of food in the refrigerator.
• Never refreeze thawed food.

| MAXIMUM FREEZING TIMES FOR FOOD FOR BABIES | |
|---|---|
| Fish | 3 months |
| Meat | 3 months |
| Poultry | 3 months |
| Fruit | 3 months |
| Vegetables | 3 months |
| Soups | 3 months |
| Breads & cakes | 3 months |

## Reheating and microwaving

Your freezer and microwave oven are invaluable when planning and making food for young children.

When reheating food for your baby, remember that babies do not like hot food. If food has been refrigerated or frozen, it should be briefly brought to a boil then cooled to lukewarm before serving. Freshly made food can be reheated over a saucepan of gently simmering water or in a microwave oven.

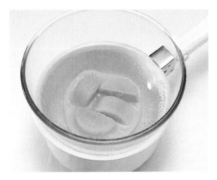

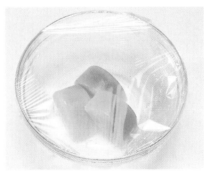

While the microwave is a great timesaver when cooking and reheating baby food, great care must be taken. Microwaved food continues to cook after being removed from the oven and can therefore be very hot.

Never serve food cooked or reheated in a microwave oven before stirring and then testing it.

Pause to stir food at intervals during microwave reheating to allow for even heat distribution.

Allow microwaved food to rest outside the oven for several minutes before feeding it to your baby.

## FOOD INTOLERANCE AND ALLERGIES

Food intolerance occurs when food is not digested properly, such as gluten intolerance (known as celiac disease) or milk (lactose) intolerance. A very small number of babies can also suffer true allergic reactions to certain foods.

Symptoms of allergy or intolerance can include swelling and itching around the mouth or throat, diarrhea, stomach pain, vomiting, runny nose, coughing, eczema, hives, hay fever or asthma. But since most children will exhibit at least some of these symptoms during their infancy, whether they are allergic or not, you should seek medical advice, if you think your baby has a problem. It is important to establish whether there actually *is* an allergy as you might be needlessly eliminating a useful food from the baby's diet.

A tendency to allergy can be hereditary so, if you or your immediate family have a history of food reactions, such as asthma, hay fever, eczema or a reaction to peanuts, you should proceed more cautiously when introducing solids. However, most small children will grow out of their allergy and often, if there is a reaction, it can be very mild.

Eggs, peanuts, cow's milk, wheat, shellfish, strawberries and artificial colorings are the foods most commonly linked to allergic reactions and intolerance, so you should not offer these foods until baby is a certain age: avoid cow's milk (except infant formula) and wheat products for the first 6 months; avoid egg white and strawberries before 9 to 12 months; leave peanut products until baby is 12 months old (or 5 years if a close relative is allergic). When first adding them to the diet, do so one at a time and in small amounts – if you notice a reaction, wait a month before trying the food again or seek medical advice.

# 4 to 6 months
## WHERE TO BEGIN

As a general guide, you should start to think about introducing solid food between four and six months if . . .

• Your breastfeeding baby is no longer putting on as much weight as he should, despite your efforts to increase supply.

• Your bottle-fed baby is not satisfied with the usual amounts of formula and constantly seems hungry and unsettled.

• Your baby is now six months old and is still fully milk fed.

If you are in any doubt about when to introduce solids, consult your doctor or early-childhood nurse.

### starting solids

Initially, solid food should be offered *after* the breast or bottle feeding, as milk is still the major source of nourishment. Alternatively, offer half milk feeding, then solid food. This will take the edge off baby's hunger, but he will still be interested in what you have to offer and will be more relaxed and settled. Finish with the remainder of the familiar milk feeding.

Traditionally, the first food to be offered is rice cereal as it is well tolerated, but you can also start with a little pureed fruit or veggies instead, or mashed ripe banana or avocado.

If starting with rice cereal, mix 1 to 2 teaspoons with 1/2 to 1 ounce expressed breast milk, prepared formula or cooled, boiled water until it is a thin paste consistency. Using a spoon without sharp edges (the bowl and spoon do not need to be sterilized), offer baby 1 to 2 teaspoons of the cereal mix at the feeding of the day you prefer. Hold the spoon to his lips and allow him to suck the cereal off. Do not push the spoon back into his mouth, it will cause him to gag. Take your time – remember that up until now, your baby has sucked his food, so having a spoon in his mouth is a very new sensation. Repeat this process once a day for a few days.

2  If this step was a success, you can now offer cereal twice a day, for several days, gradually increasing the amount and thickening the consistency to suit your baby, until he is eating up to 1 1/2 to 3 tablespoons at a time.

If he consistently refuses the cereal (it *is* a bit like wallpaper paste, after all), then try something else. If he refuses this as well, give up for a week or so, continue with milk only, then try again. Stay calm – and remind yourself there are very few fully milk-fed adults!

3  Next, add a small amount of pureed, stewed apple, pear or very ripe mashed banana to rice cereal. Gradually increase the puree over several days until you are serving equal amounts of cereal and fruit. If this is well tolerated, you can vary one meal by introducing pureed vegetables, usually potato, pumpkin and carrot to start. Offer 1 to 2 teaspoons, slowly increasing the amount over several days to 3 to 4 1/2 tablespoons.

4  Gradually increase the variety of vegetables and other foods to allow baby to become accustomed to new tastes and textures. Introduce new foods one at a time and allow a few days on each new food to ensure that baby has no adverse reaction to it, before starting the next.

5  If baby is happily eating two "meals", then you can gradually add a third, so that he is eventually eating 3 to 4 1/2 tablespoons of food, three times a day.

## pureed apple or pear

**1 medium apple or 1 small pear, peeled, cored, chopped**

Boil, steam or microwave apple or pear until tender; drain over small bowl, reserving 1 1/2 tablespoons cooking liquid. Blend or process fruit with cooking liquid or boiled water until smooth.

MAKES 1/2 CUP

**Storage**  Covered, in refrigerator, up to 2 days
**Freeze**  Suitable, in individual portions

☺ TIP  Mix a little of this pureed fruit with yogurt.

## pureed potato or pumpkin

**1/2 cup peeled and chopped potato or pumpkin**

Boil, steam or microwave potato or pumpkin until tender; drain. Blend or process with enough breast milk, formula or cooled boiled water until of desired consistency.

MAKES 1/2 CUP

**Storage**  Covered, in refrigerator, up to 2 days
**Freeze**  Suitable, in individual portions

☺ TIP  Mashed avocado is an excellent choice for one of your baby's first foods; it is also good blended with a little of the pureed pear or apple.

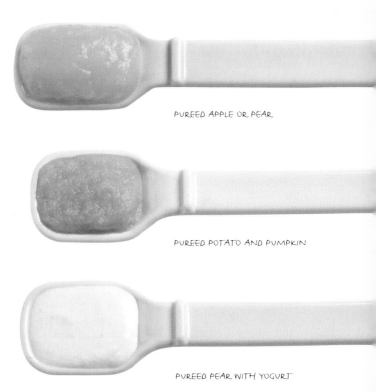

PUREED APPLE OR PEAR

PUREED POTATO AND PUMPKIN

PUREED PEAR WITH YOGURT

## Introducing different foods

As your baby grows, so should the number of different foods being offered. If he fusses when given a particular food for the first time, leave it for a while and continue with foods that have already been accepted. But do keep trying new foods at frequent intervals.

You are not, however, running a restaurant for infant gourmands, providing a new taste sensation at every meal! Young babies do not get bored eating the same things repeatedly because they have no prior knowledge about different flavors or textures. This is also true of salt – the taste for salt is acquired. Although you might think the food tastes bland, your baby will not think this and you should not add any salt to food that you prepare for babies under 12 months – excessive sodium has the potential to damage immature kidneys.

Sugar should also be used sparingly – for the sake of your baby's health, you do not want to encourage a "sweet tooth".

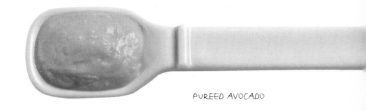

PUREED AVOCADO

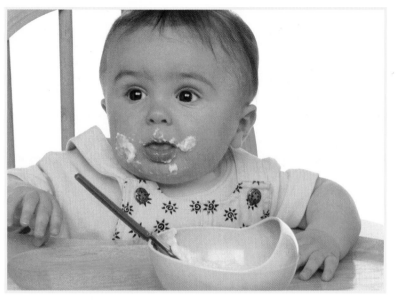

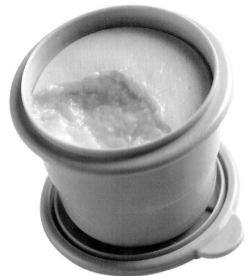

VANILLA PUDDING

## photostop

It is fun to record baby's first mouthful for posterity. Some babies seem to understand immediately what they are supposed to do, swallow happily and look at you expectantly for more, like a baby bird. Others react as though you have taken an enormous liberty and get a "you must be joking" look that is definitely one for the album!

## vanilla pudding

**1 1/2 tablespoons cornstarch**
**2/3 cup formula or breast milk**
**2 teaspoons sugar**
**1/4 teaspoon vanilla extract**

Blend cornstarch with 1 1/2 tablespoons of the milk in a small bowl until smooth. Bring remaining milk to boil in small pan; remove from heat. Add sugar, vanilla and cornstarch mixture, stirring over heat until mixture boils and thickens. Pour vanilla pudding into small bowl, cover; refrigerate several hours or until set.

MAKES 2/3 CUP

**Storage**  Covered, in refrigerator, up to 2 days

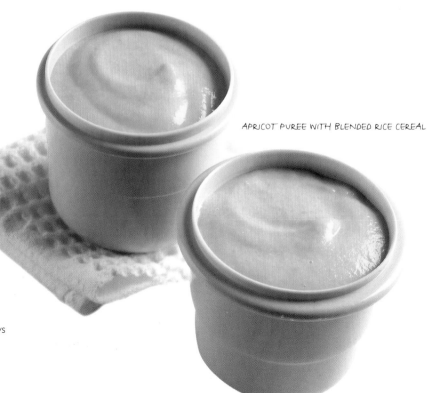

APRICOT PUREE WITH BLENDED RICE CEREAL

## apricot puree with blended rice cereal

**2/3 cup dried apricots**
**1 1/2 cups water**
**3 tablespoons blended cereal**
**1/3 cup formula or breast milk, warmed**

Combine apricots and water in small pan; simmer, covered, about 20 minutes or until apricots are tender. Blend apricots and cooking liquid until smooth.

Mix cereal in small bowl with breast milk or formula; serve topped with 1 1/2 tablespoons apricot puree.

PUREE MAKES 1 1/4 CUPS

**Storage**  Puree, covered, in refrigerator up to 2 days
**Freeze**  Puree, suitable in individual portions

## *food intolerance*

As a small number of babies find it difficult to digest **gluten** (found in wheat products), it is best to avoid this in the first 6 months. That is why we start with rice cereal — although soy, corn, seed tapioca and tapioca are also suitable.

**Egg white** can also occasionally cause an adverse reaction so it is best to avoid eggs until 9 to 12 months.

### apple cream of wheat

**1 tablespoon cream of wheat**
**¹/₃ cup cooled boiled water**
**¹/₃ cup apple juice**

Combine all ingredients in small pan; simmer, uncovered, about 2 minutes or until thickened slightly.
MAKES ²/₃ CUP
**Storage**  Covered, in refrigerator, up to 2 days

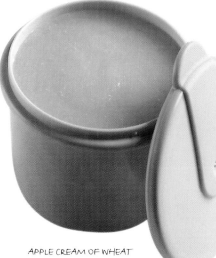

APPLE CREAM OF WHEAT

### ricotta with pear puree

**¹/₃ cup ricotta cheese**
**3 tablespoons pureed pear**

Push ricotta through a fine sieve. Mix ricotta in small bowl with pureed pear until smooth. Add a little extra breast milk or cooled boiled water if necessary.
MAKES ¹/₂ CUP
**Storage**  Covered, in refrigerator, up to 2 days

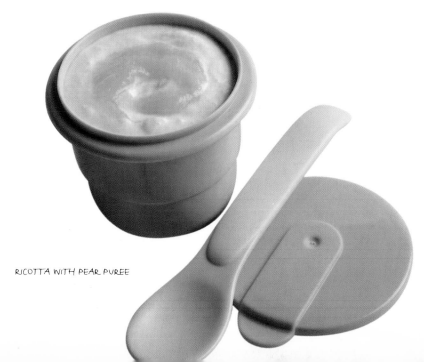

RICOTTA WITH PEAR PUREE

### PREPARED BABY FOODS

Commercial baby foods are useful "convenience" foods when traveling or in an emergency, and can be used on their own or in conjunction with homemade foods. They are quick to prepare, safe and the range is extensive; however, they are often less economical than the foods you make yourself and tend to provide less variety in texture and taste.

• Always check labels before purchasing commercial baby foods so that you are fully aware of their contents.

• Discard any remaining portions of commercial baby food if your child has been fed directly from the container.

• If you know beforehand that all the food will not be eaten, spoon a single serving from the container and heat it separately. The remaining food, covered tightly, can be refrigerated for up to 2 days.

• Commercial baby food in glass jars can be reheated in a saucepan half-filled with boiling water or placed in your microwave oven — but always remember to remove a jar's metal lid though before reheating in a microwave.

# 6 to 9 months
## TASTE TESTING

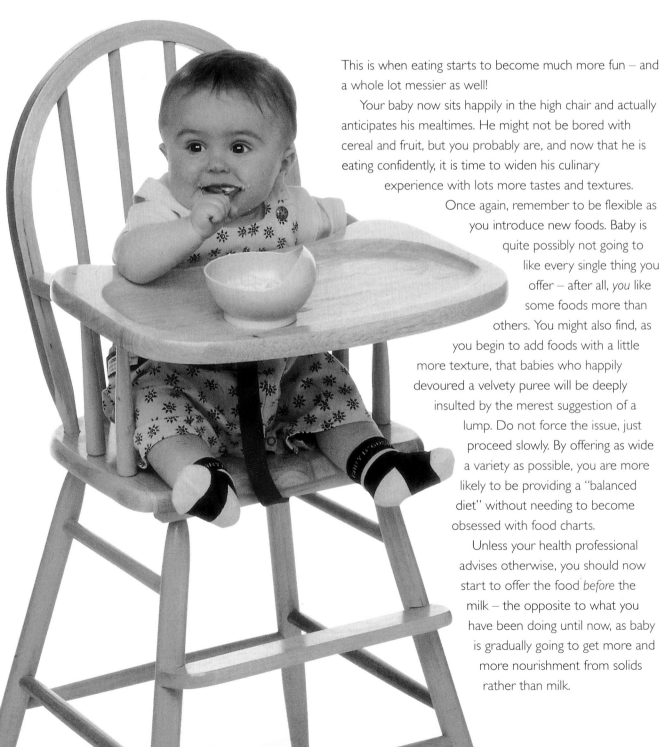

This is when eating starts to become much more fun – and a whole lot messier as well!

Your baby now sits happily in the high chair and actually anticipates his mealtimes. He might not be bored with cereal and fruit, but you probably are, and now that he is eating confidently, it is time to widen his culinary experience with lots more tastes and textures. Once again, remember to be flexible as you introduce new foods. Baby is quite possibly not going to like every single thing you offer – after all, *you* like some foods more than others. You might also find, as you begin to add foods with a little more texture, that babies who happily devoured a velvety puree will be deeply insulted by the merest suggestion of a lump. Do not force the issue, just proceed slowly. By offering as wide a variety as possible, you are more likely to be providing a "balanced diet" without needing to become obsessed with food charts.

Unless your health professional advises otherwise, you should now start to offer the food *before* the milk – the opposite to what you have been doing until now, as baby is gradually going to get more and more nourishment from solids rather than milk.

## oatmeal mush

*Best made just before mealtime, oatmeal can be served with warm or cold milk, a little maple syrup, karo syrup or pureed fruit.*

**¹/₃ cup rolled oats**
**³/₄ cup water or milk**

Combine all ingredients in small pan; bring to boil, cook, stirring, about 2 minutes or until thickened.

MAKES 1 CUP

**Microwave** Combine ingredients in microwave-safe bowl, cover; microwave on HIGH (100%) about 2 minutes or until thickened, pausing halfway during cooking time to stir.

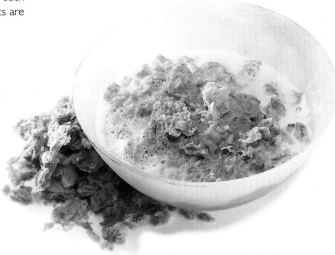

OATMEAL MUSH

## breakfast biscuits

Crush whole-wheat malted breakfast biscuits (such as Weeta-bix, Shredded Wheat etc) with enough breast milk, formula or cooled boiled water until of desired consistency.

## toast fingers

A great food for babies to suck and "chew". Toasted crusts are good, too.

## blended rice cereal combo

Try stirring pureed fruit and yogurt into blended rice cereal.

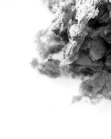

TOAST FINGERS

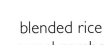

BREAKFAST BISCUITS

*Iron and your baby* From about 6 months of age, babies start to require extra iron in their diet. This is easily included if you plan to feed your baby meat, but for non meat-eating families, it can be a little more of a challenge.

Iron is present in some of the food that most babies eat (leafy greens, egg yolks, cereals, breads, beans and lentils, for instance); however, some of this iron is in a form not easily absorbed into the system.

If foods containing Vitamin C (citrus fruits, kiwi fruit, cantaloupe, tomatoes, broccoli, papaya and bell pepper) are consumed in conjunction with the foods listed earlier, absorption will be facilitated.

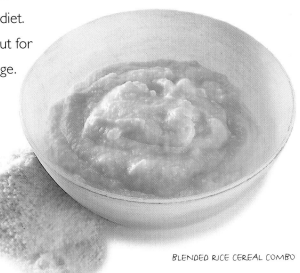

BLENDED RICE CEREAL COMBO

## pureed mixed vegetables

*Sweet potato, beans, broccoli or spinach can also be used. We have used this recipe in the others shown on this page.*

**I medium potato,
 chopped coarsely**
**I medium carrot,
 chopped coarsely**
**I medium zucchini,
 chopped coarsely**

Boil, steam or microwave vegetables until tender, drain; blend or process until smooth. If necessary, stir in a little breast milk, formula or cooled boiled water until of desired consistency.

MAKES 2 CUPS

**Storage** Covered, in refrigerator, up to 2 days
**Freeze** Suitable, in individual portions

PUREED MIXED VEGETABLES
WITH FRIED LAMB PUREE

## white or cheese sauce

*Try both versions of this sauce with pureed mixed vegetables to introduce new tastes to your baby.*

**I ¹/₂ tablespoons butter**
**2 teaspoons all-purpose flour**
 **¹/₂ cup formula or breast milk**
 **I ¹/₂ tablespoons finely
 grated cheddar cheese,
 optional**

Melt butter in small pan. Stir in flour; cook, stirring, until bubbling. Remove from heat; gradually stir in milk. Cook, stirring, until mixture boils and thickens; add cheese, if using. Stir sauce through pureed vegetables.

MAKES ¹/₂ CUP

**Storage** Covered, in refrigerator, up to 2 days

CHEESE SAUCE

## steamed fish puree

**I small fish fillet**

Remove any bones or skin from fish. Place in steamer basket; cook, covered, over pan of simmering water about 5 minutes or until cooked through. Blend or process with a little breast milk, formula or cooled boiled water until of desired consistency. Serve with pureed green vegetables.

MAKES ABOUT ¹/₂ CUP

**Storage** Covered, in refrigerator, up to 2 days
**Freeze** Suitable, in individual portions

## fried lamb puree

*Any lean lamb, from a small fillet or trimmed from a leg, or lean beef can be used for this recipe.*

**¹/₂ teaspoon olive oil**
**I lamb chop, trimmed**

Heat oil in small pan, cook lamb until browned both sides and cooked through. When cool enough to handle, remove meat from bone; blend or process with a little breast milk, formula or cooled boiled water until smooth. Serve with pureed vegetables, if desired.

MAKES ¹/₄ CUP

**Storage** Covered, in refrigerator up to 2 days
**Freeze** Suitable, in individual portions

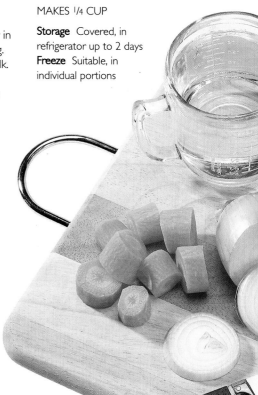

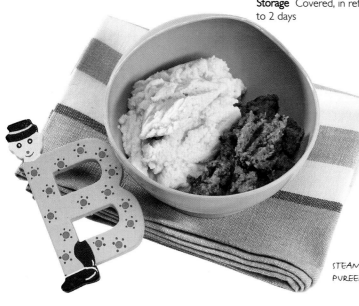

STEAMED FISH PUREE WITH
PUREED GREEN VEGETABLES

## chicken stock

*Omit the chicken and you will have a healthy and tasty vegetable stock good for soups and sauces, or for thinning purees.*

- **1 lb chicken bones**
- **3 trimmed celery stalks, chopped**
- **2 medium carrots, chopped**
- **1 medium yellow onion, chopped**
- **1 sprig parsley**
- **1 bay leaf**
- **2 quarts or 8 cups water**

Combine all ingredients in large pan; simmer, uncovered, 1 hour. Strain into large bowl; discard bones and vegetables. Refrigerate stock overnight. Remove and discard solidified fat from the surface. If stock is to be kept longer, it is best to freeze it in small quantities. When reheating stock, be sure to bring it to the boil before using.

MAKES 6 CUPS

**Storage** Covered, in refrigerator, up to 2 days
**Freeze** Suitable, in individual portions

TIP Great finger food A cooked and cooled lamb rib chop bone makes a great treat for an older baby to suck and "chew" on.

## chicken and vegetable soup

- **2 chicken thighs (14 oz)**
- **1 quart or 4 cups chicken stock (at left)**
- **1 small yellow onion, chopped**
- **1 medium carrot, chopped**
- **1 trimmed celery stalk, chopped**
- **1 small potato, chopped**
- **3 tablespoons barley**

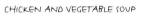

CHICKEN AND VEGETABLE SOUP

Remove fat from chicken. Place chicken and stock in medium pan, bring to boil; simmer, uncovered, 30 minutes. Strain over large bowl; reserve chicken and cooking liquid. Remove meat from chicken thighs; discard bones. Return chicken, liquid, vegetables and barley to same pan; simmer, uncovered, about 15 minutes or until barley is tender. Blend or process, in batches, until just smooth.

MAKES 4 CUPS

**Storage** Covered, in refrigerator, up to 2 days
**Freeze** Suitable, in individual portions
*Rice or pasta can be substituted for barley in this recipe.*

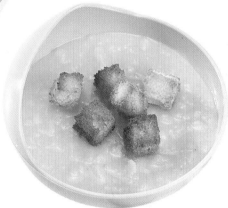

POTATO SOUP

## potato soup

- **3 medium potatoes, chopped**
- **3 cups chicken (or vegetable) stock**

Place potatoes in medium pan with stock; bring to boil. Simmer, covered, about 15 minutes or until potatoes are tender. Blend or process, in batches, until smooth. Serve, topped with toast cubes for older babies, if desired.

MAKES 4 CUPS

**Storage** Covered, in refrigerator, up to 2 days. Reheat as required, thinning if necessary with a little stock, formula or breast milk
**Freeze** Suitable, in individual portions

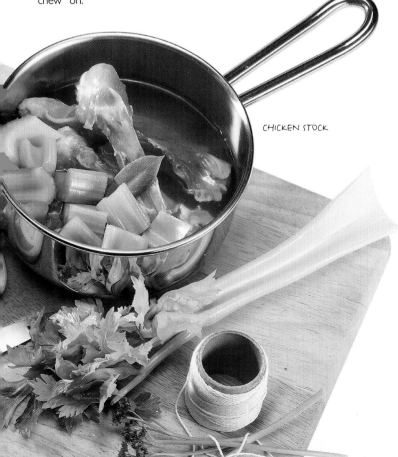

CHICKEN STOCK

## lamb shank broth

- **1 lamb shank, trimmed**
- **1 medium potato, chopped coarsely**
- **1 medium carrot, chopped coarsely**
- **1 trimmed celery stalk, chopped coarsely**
- **1 1/2 tablespoons barley**
- **4 cups water**

Place all ingredients in medium pan; bring to boil. Simmer, covered, about 1 hour or until meat is tender. When cool enough to handle, remove lamb shank from pan; remove meat from shank, discard bone. Blend or process meat with vegetables and cooking liquid, in batches, until soup is almost smooth.

MAKES 4 CUPS

**Storage** Covered, in refrigerator, up to 2 days
**Freeze** Suitable, in individual portions

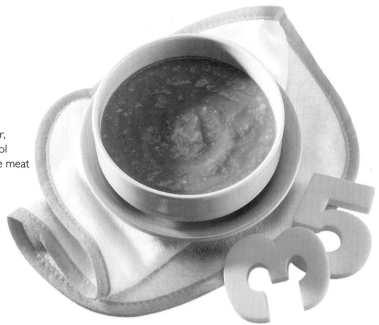

LAMB SHANK BROTH

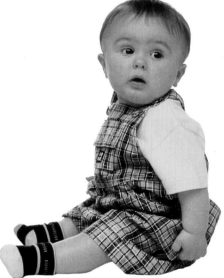

*foods to avoid at this stage*

Because they have been known to cause adverse reactions in a small number of babies, **honey, peanut products** and **strawberries** should all be avoided until baby is at least 12 months old. **Egg white** should also be delayed until 9 to 12 months.

## zucchini and corn pasta

*Elbow macaroni can be substituted for orzo.*

- **1 1/2 tablespoons butter**
- **1 small tomato, chopped finely**
- **1 small zucchini, grated coarsely**
- **1/3 cup orzo**
- **3 tablespoons creamed corn**

Melt butter in small pan; cook tomato and zucchini, stirring, until vegetables are tender. Meanwhile, cook orzo in medium pan of boiling water, uncovered, until tender; drain. Combine warm orzo and vegetable mixture with corn in small bowl.

MAKES ABOUT 2 CUPS

**Storage** Covered, in refrigerator, up to 2 days
**Freeze** Suitable, in individual portions

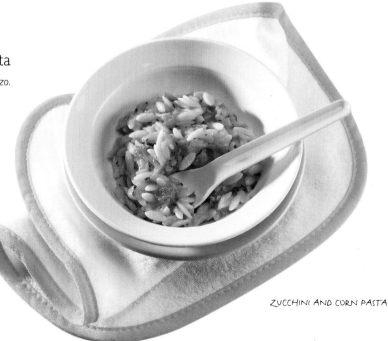

ZUCCHINI AND CORN PASTA

## stewed fruit compote

**2 cups water**
**¹/₃ cup dried apricots**
**¹/₃ cup pitted prunes**
**I small pear, peeled, quartered, sliced thickly**
**I cinnamon stick**
**I ¹/₂ tablespoons brown sugar**

Combine all ingredients in medium pan; simmer, covered, about 20 minutes or until pears are tender. Cool; discard cinnamon stick. Serve mashed, with yogurt, if desired.

MAKES ABOUT 2 CUPS

**Storage** Covered, in refrigerator, up to 2 days

**Freeze** Suitable, in individual portions

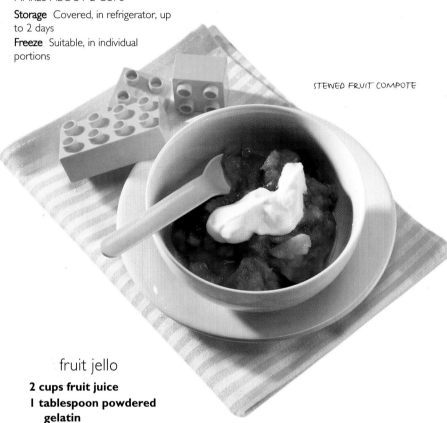

STEWED FRUIT COMPOTE

## fruit jello

**2 cups fruit juice**
**I tablespoon powdered gelatin**

Place ¹/4 cup of the juice in a cup; sprinkle gelatin over juice. Stand cup in small pan of simmering water, stir until gelatin is dissolved. Stir gelatin mixture into remaining juice in medium bowl; refrigerate until firm.

FRUIT JELLO

## daily meal plan

This plan only includes 3 breast- or bottle-feedings. Often young babies are still on 4 or 5 milk feedings, so continue with these feedings within this plan in a way that works for you and your baby. Lunch and dinner suggestions are interchangeable. Times are merely a guide.

EARLY MORNING
6am     Breast or bottle

BREAKFAST
8am     Oatmeal mush or
        shredded wheat
        Toast fingers
        Diluted juice

MORNING SNACK
10am    Yogurt and fruit
        Water/diluted juice

LUNCH
12.30pm Creamy vegetable
        puree
        Breast or bottle

AFTERNOON SNACK
3pm     Mashed banana
        Water/diluted juice

DINNER
5.30pm  Lamb shank broth
        Fruit Jello
        Breast or bottle

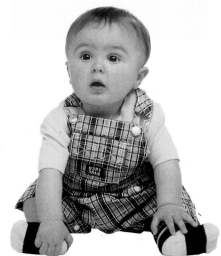

# 9 to 12 months
## GREATER VARIETY

The greatest change around now is that your baby probably has teeth, making finger food a new option. But do not think that a lack of teeth means she cannot have finger food – her little gums are hard enough to deal with a variety of foods. Your baby will probably love finger food – not only does it offer a whole new range of interesting tastes and textures, it also gives her a measure of control that appeals to her newly developing sense of independence. You will also find that finger food provides a marvelous distraction from playing pat-a-cake with the rest of her meal. At this stage, it is only going to be a temporary distraction and despite the fact that mealtimes can end with both of you looking as though you have been rolling in the dish of the day, it is important to let your baby experiment with her food. Those inquisitive little fingers will eventually transfer some of the meal into her mouth! Her enthusiasm is more important than your kitchen floor – if she wants to have the spoon, give her one of her own; this is the first step to learning to feed herself, after all.

### Helping fussy eaters to eat

Some babies can be very contrary when it comes to food, even those who started as textbook eaters. Try not to worry if food is refused – your baby is not going to starve! She may simply have begun to work out that her refusal to eat produces interesting results – lots of attention, for a start.

• Do not allow babies to eat or drink too much between mealtimes – this can lead to refusing meals. On the other hand, if the small-and-often form of eating is mutually acceptable, food eaten as a snack is just as nutritious as the same food eaten at specific "mealtimes".

• Experiment with different flavors, textures and combinations, but do not impose *your* idea of a suitable combination on the baby – if she wants to dip a chop bone in her bread and butter pudding, then who cares?

• If your fussy eater will only eat one favorite food, there is nothing wrong with serving it up repeatedly. Offer alternatives but do not get upset if they are refused.

• Try to keep it a happy time (no matter how stressed you feel) – a story or song can occasionally help, but do not feel you have to put on *Showboat* either, or draw faces or fly aeroplanes with every mouthful: it is not dinner and a show! Allow the meal to end when she indicates she has had enough and resist the temptation to turn cartwheels in order to encourage a few last mouthfuls. It is a rare child who will not grasp the opportunity to see you do it again and again, then demand somersaults as well!

## muesli

*We used dried apples, apricots and currants in this version but try experimenting with raisins, dried peaches or dates to find your baby's particular likes and dislikes.*

**1 shredded wheat biscuit, crushed**
**1/4 cup bran flakes**
**1/4 cup rice crispies**
**1/2 cup your choice dried fruit, chopped finely**
**2 teaspoons dried coconut**

Combine all ingredients in medium bowl. Serve with formula, breast milk or yogurt and chopped fresh fruit, if desired.

MAKES 1 1/2 CUPS

**Storage** Airtight container, up to 1 week

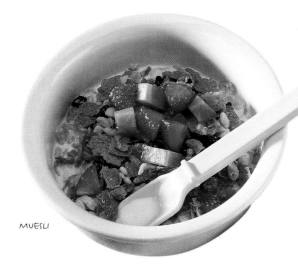

MUESLI

## mini pancakes

**1 cup self-rising flour**
**3 tablespoons superfine sugar**
**1 egg, beaten lightly**
**3/4 cup milk, approximately**

Combine flour and sugar in medium bowl; gradually whisk in egg and enough milk to make a thick, smooth batter. Drop dessertspoons of mixture into greased heavy-bottomed pan; cook until bubbles begin to appear on surface of mini pancake, turn, brown other side. Serve with yogurt and stewed or pureed fruit, if desired, or a drizzle of maple syrup.

MAKES ABOUT 20

**Storage** Airtight container, up to 2 days

MINI PANCAKES

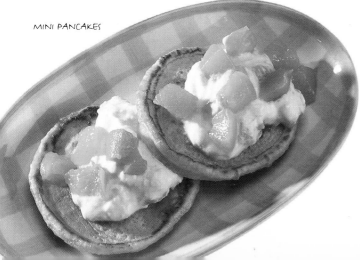

## homemade zwieback

**1 loaf unsliced bread**

Trim crusts from all sides and ends of loaf. Cut bread into 5/8-inch slices; cut slices into 5/8-inch fingers. Place on baking sheets, bake at 250°F about 1 hour or until bread is dried and crisp.

MAKES ABOUT 70

**Storage** Airtight container, up to 1 week

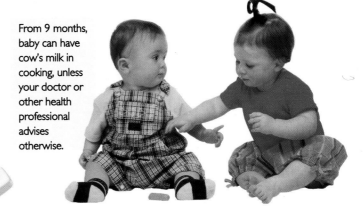

From 9 months, baby can have cow's milk in cooking, unless your doctor or other health professional advises otherwise.

## fruit muffins

**2 cups self-rising flour**
**1 teaspoon apple-pie spice**
**1/2 cup firmly packed brown sugar**
**1/2 cup golden raisins**
**1 cup milk**
**5/8 cup butter, melted**
**1 egg, beaten lightly**

Grease three 12-cup small (3-tablespoon-capacity) muffin pans. Combine flour, spice, sugar and golden raisins in large bowl. Stir in milk, butter and egg; do not overmix (batter should be coarse and slightly lumpy). Divide mixture among muffin tin cups; bake muffins at 400°F about 15 minutes or until browned.

MAKES 36

**Storage** Airtight container, up to 2 days
**Freeze** Suitable

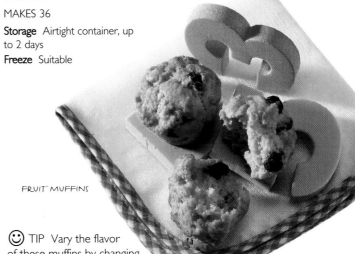

FRUIT MUFFINS

☺ TIP Vary the flavor of these muffins by changing the dried fruit to either chopped dried apricots, raisins, pitted dates or pitted prunes, or a combination of any of these.

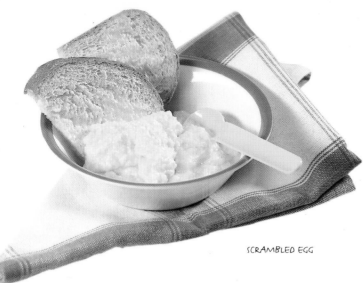

SCRAMBLED EGG

## scrambled egg

**1 egg**
**1 ½ tablespoons milk**
**1 teaspoon butter**

Whisk egg and milk in small bowl. Heat butter in small pan, add egg mixture; cook over low heat, stirring gently, until egg just sets. Serve with buttered bread.

☺ TIP  Make scrambled egg just before serving. Remember that this cannot be fed to children who have not yet successfully included egg in their diet.

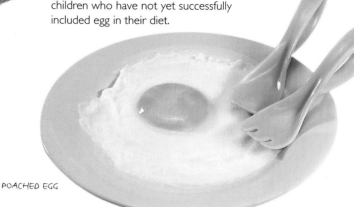

POACHED EGG

## poached egg

Break 1 egg into small shallow pan of gently simmering water, turn off heat, place lid on pan; stand about 3 minutes or until egg white is just set. Remove with slotted spoon or egg slide, serve immediately.

## *daily meal plan*

EARLY MORNING
6am      Breast or bottle

BREAKFAST
8am      Muesli
         Toast fingers
         Diluted juice

MORNING SNACK
10am     Muffin
         Water/diluted juice

LUNCH
12.30pm  Chopped tomato
         and bread
         Breast or bottle

AFTERNOON SNACK
3pm      Mashed banana
         Water/diluted juice

DINNER
5.30pm   Chicken and
         vegetable soup
         Egg custard
         Breast
         or bottle

## avocado dip

**½ ripe avocado**
**¼ cup finely grated cheddar cheese**
**1 ½ tablespoons finely chopped tomato**
**1 teaspoon yogurt**

Blend, process or mash all ingredients in small bowl. Serve with blanched vegetable sticks for older children or as a meal for younger babies.

MAKES ½ CUP
*Best made just before serving*

## chopped tomato and bread

A delicious light meal for an older baby. Toss chopped buttered bread, crusts removed, with chopped skinned and seeded tomato in small bowl; add a little grated cheese, cottage cheese or chopped ham, as desired.

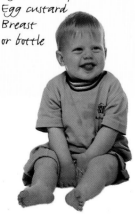

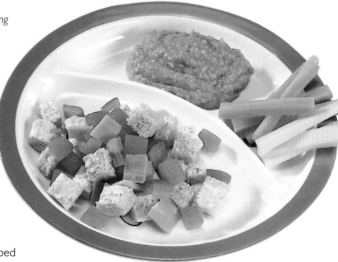

CHOPPED TOMATO AND BREAD
WITH AVOCADO DIP

## bread and butter pudding

**2 slices white bread, crusts removed**
**butter**
**1 1/4 cups milk**
**2 eggs**
**1 1/2 tablespoons superfine sugar**
**1/4 teaspoon vanilla extract**
**pinch ground nutmeg**

Spread bread lightly with butter; cut into small triangle-shaped pieces. Divide bread among four 1/2 cup greased heatproof dishes; place dishes in baking dish. Whisk milk, eggs, sugar and vanilla in medium bowl; pour egg mixture over bread, sprinkle with nutmeg. Pour enough boiling water into baking dish to come halfway up sides of dishes. Bake, uncovered, at 350°F about 20 minutes or until puddings are just set.

MAKES 4 SERVINGS

**Storage** Covered, in refrigerator, up to 2 days

☺ TIP **Stirred custard** You can make a plain stirred custard easily by beating the same quantities of eggs and sugar shown above together, in the top half of a double saucepan or small heatproof bowl, until mixture starts to thicken, then whisking in the same amounts of warmed milk and vanilla. Place pan or bowl over top of a larger pan half-filled with simmering water; cook, stirring, until custard is thick enough to coat the back of a spoon. Be careful not to overheat the custard or allow water to touch base of pan as custard could curdle. Remove from heat and larger pan as soon as the custard has thickened.

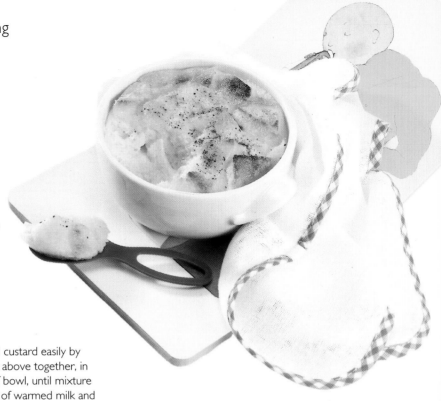

BREAD AND BUTTER PUDDING

## quick creamed rice

**1/2 cup (125ml) milk**
**2 teaspoons brown sugar**
**1/4 cup cooked short grain rice**

Combine milk and sugar in small pan; bring to boil, stir in rice. Cook, stirring, about 5 minutes or until thickened. Serve topped with fruit, if desired.

MAKES 1 SERVING

**Storage** Covered, in refrigerator, up to 2 days

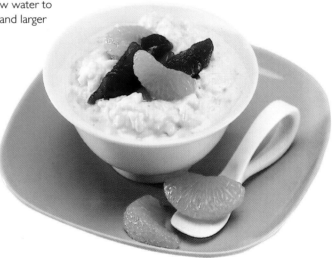

QUICK CREAMED RICE

## sweet couscous

**3/4 cup milk**
**1 1/2 tablespoons couscous**
**1 teaspoon sugar**
**pinch ground cinnamon**

Combine all ingredients in small pan; simmer, stirring, about 12 minutes or until thickened.
Serve with sliced banana, if desired.

MAKES 1 SERVING

**Storage** Covered, in refrigerator, up to 2 days

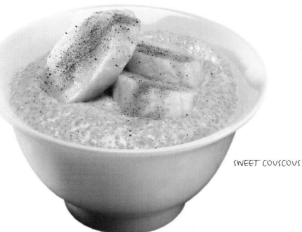

SWEET COUSCOUS

# 12 to 18 months
## BITE-SIZE BITS

By the beginning of the second year, your toddler will probably be ready to share quite a number of the foods you serve to the rest of the family – the goal is in sight! However, all children vary in their development. At this age, some are adventurous with their tastes while others are totally uninterested in the whole business. Some will only eat if they can feed themselves, while others still absolutely insist on being spoon-fed every mouthful. This should not really come as a surprise – just like adults, children's tastes and the size of their appetites vary with each individual.

That is why our menus are only guidelines, not rules, and flexibility is still the key to retaining your sanity and sense of humor. If your toddler thinks scrambled eggs are beyond the pale, whip the egg into a custard instead – it has the same nutritional value.

Children who are already walking will tend to use up more energy and might be hungrier than their less-mobile counterparts. If your child is at the stage where he needs extra food and is feeding himself quite competently – taking bite-size pieces, then chewing and swallowing before putting more in his mouth – you can now introduce more advanced meals.

For those babies whose tastes are still rather conservative, you will need to proceed slowly as you add new tastes and textures. It is important however, to foster independence – instead of simply spooning the food into his mouth, place a filled spoon in his hand and let him take it to his mouth himself. This reinforces the idea that he is the one making the decisions about eating and with all the magnificent perversity of the one-year-old mind, this might help to make him more adventurous about what he eats!

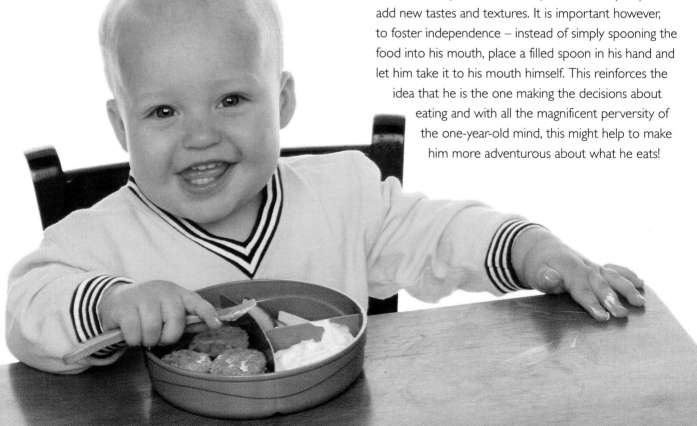

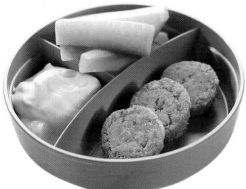

MINI LENTIL PATTIES

## stuffed baby potatoes

A quick and tasty meal for young toddlers. Bake, boil, steam or microwave new potatoes until tender; drain. Halve potatoes; scoop out a third of the flesh then trim bottoms so they set flat. Combine potato flesh with a filling of your choice and spoon into potatoes. Try your toddler with some of the following flavors:

• mashed boiled egg mixed with a dollop of low-fat mayonnaise

• mashed avocado with finely chopped ham

• baked beans

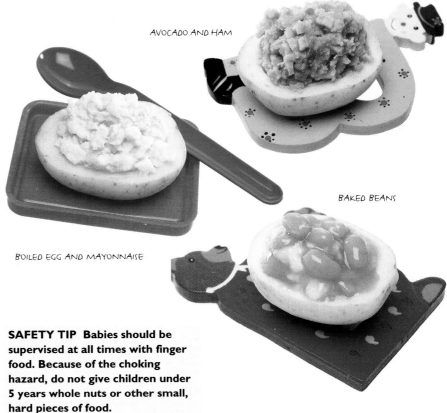

AVOCADO AND HAM

BAKED BEANS

BOILED EGG AND MAYONNAISE

## mini lentil patties

**¼ cup red lentils**

**7 oz coarsely chopped orange sweet potato**

**3 tablespoons finely chopped celery**

**¼ cup coarsely grated apple**

**½ clove garlic, crushed**

**¼ cup fresh breadcrumbs**

**½ cup packaged breadcrumbs**

Add lentils to small pan of boiling water; boil, uncovered, about 10 minutes or until tender, drain. Meanwhile, boil, steam or microwave orange sweet potato until tender; drain, mash until smooth.

Combine lentils and orange sweet potato in small bowl with celery, apple, garlic and fresh breadcrumbs; shape rounded tablespoons of mixture into patties. Coat patties in packaged breadcrumbs; place on oiled baking sheet, spray lightly with cooking-oil spray. Bake at 350°F 15 minutes or until browned lightly.

MAKES 16 PATTIES

**Storage** Covered, in refrigerator, up to 2 days

**Freeze** Suitable

**SAFETY TIP Babies should be supervised at all times with finger food. Because of the choking hazard, do not give children under 5 years whole nuts or other small, hard pieces of food.**

## spinach and ricotta ravioli with buttered crumbs

*Introduce various other filled pastas to your toddler.*

**⅔ cup ravioli filled with spinach and ricotta**

**2 teaspoons butter**

**¼ cup fresh breadcrumbs**

Add ravioli to medium pan of boiling water; boil, uncovered, until tender, drain. Meanwhile, melt butter in small pan, add breadcrumbs; cook, stirring, until browned lightly. Toss breadcrumbs through ravioli.

MAKES 1 SERVING

*Best made just before serving*

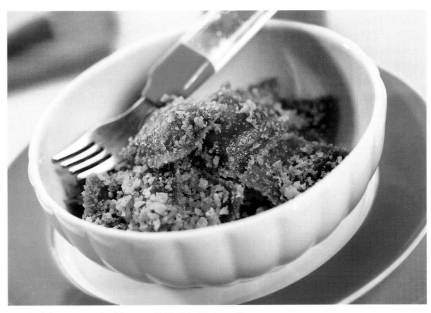

SPINACH AND RICOTTA RAVIOLI WITH BUTTERED CRUMBS

# *daily meal plan*

**EARLY MORNING**
6am   Breast or milk

**BREAKFAST**
8am   Scrambled egg
with toast fingers
Fresh fruit or juice

**MORNING SNACK**
10am   Yogurt or cheese
snack

**LUNCH**
12.30pm   Corn and broccoli
florets
Breast or bottle

**AFTERNOON SNACK**
3pm   Banana fruit ice
Water/ juice

**DINNER**
5.30pm   Mini lentil patties
with chopped tomato
and avocado
Jello
Breast or bottle

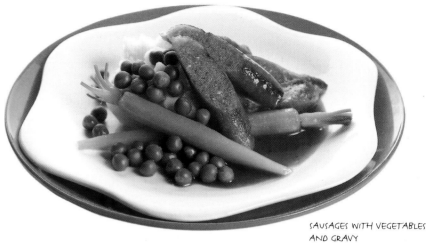

SAUSAGES WITH VEGETABLES
AND GRAVY

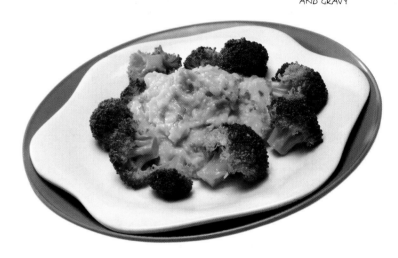

CORN AND BROCCOLI FLORETS

## sausages with vegetables and gravy

**2 thin beef sausages (5 oz)**
**¼ cup frozen peas**
**4 baby carrots**
**1 medium potato, chopped coarsely**
**1 teaspoon butter**
**3 tablespoons milk**
**2 teaspoons powdered gravy mix**
**½ cup water**

Cook sausages on heated oiled griddle (or broiler or barbecue) until browned all over and cooked as desired; cover to keep warm.

Boil, steam or microwave vegetables, separately, until tender; drain. Mash potatoes with butter and milk until smooth. Combine gravy mix and water in small pan; cook, stirring, until gravy boils and thickens. Simmer, uncovered, 2 minutes.

MAKES 2 SERVINGS

**Storage**  Covered, separately, in refrigerator, up to 2 days
**Freeze**  Uncooked sausages suitable

## corn and broccoli florets

**1 slice bacon, chopped finely**
**½ cup canned creamed corn**
**1 cup broccoli florets**

Heat medium pan; cook bacon, stirring, until crisp, drain on paper towels.

Heat corn in medium pan; add bacon, cook until hot.

Boil, steam or microwave broccoli until tender; drain. Place corn and bacon mixture in center of plate; arrange broccoli around corn.

MAKES 2 SERVINGS

**Storage**  Covered, in refrigerator, up to 2 days

PASTA SHELLS WITH CHOPPED HAM, AVOCADO
AND TOMATO

## pasta shells

Toss pre-cooked pasta shells or other pasta shapes with a combination of any or all of the following, served warm or cold: cottage cheese, grated cheese, chopped tomato, chopped avocado or chopped ham. This makes delicious fingerfood even though a bit messy!

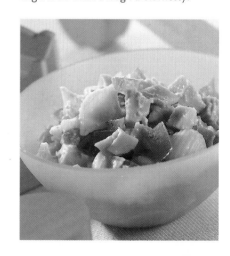

## jello

Use a packet of Jello to prepare an all-time favorite – follow the manufacturer's instructions. Alternatively, use fresh fruit juice in place of the water, and stir in freshly chopped fruit (avoid pineapple as it prevents the Jello from setting).

## banana fruit ice

This is a deliciously healthy ice cream substitute that can be served as a snack or dessert.

Mash 1 ripe medium banana in small bowl; divide banana between two small freezer-safe containers. Cover; freeze several hours or overnight. Just before serving, remove from freezer; let stand 5 minutes. Using a fork, beat banana until light-colored and creamy.

MAKES 2 SERVINGS

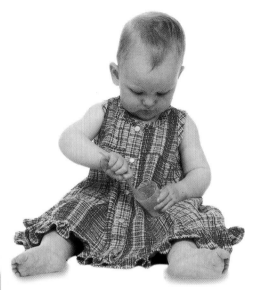

JELLO

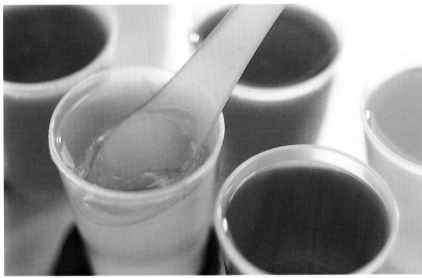

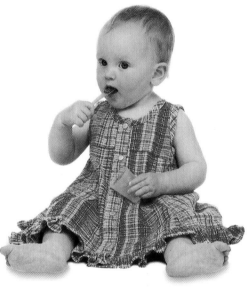

BANANA FRUIT ICE

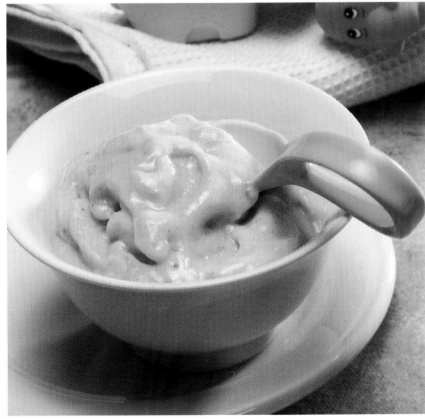

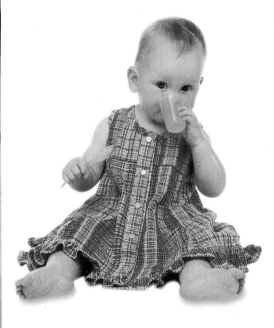

# 2 to 3 years
## QUICK AND EASY MEALS

Anyone who has had a close encounter with a two-year-old knows that occasionally it is nearly impossible to avoid losing your cool at mealtimes. On the one hand, you have a little person who is now able to eat almost anything the rest of the family eats, as well as feed himself with a considerable degree of dexterity. On the other hand, you have the average two-year-old – quixotic, willful, capricious and alert to even the slightest signal that this eating business might matter to you. Do not be drawn into the game – if food is refused, remove it without a fuss.

It might sound silly, but try to think like a two-year-old. He is insatiably curious and loves to "help". Find a small, safe task that will involve the child in the meal preparation. If he has had a hand in the preparation, he might be more inclined to eat it.

Piling large amounts of food onto the plate can also be very repugnant – just think what it must look like! Keep the serving toddler-sized and arrange it attractively – you know yourself how important presentation can be to your enjoyment of a meal. You do not have to go to the trouble of making a funny face out of everything you serve, but keep it varied and appealing . . . and small.

Serve food that you know your child enjoys. Do not worry if it is almost the same meal every night – it does not matter. Try to find substitutes for food that is disliked rather than having a battle of wills over the hated item. For instance, if he loathes veggies, serve fruit; if milk offends, try cheese or yogurt; if he hates chewing meat, offer protein that is easier to chew, such as ground meat, chicken or fish.

And on the days when you are starting to feel completely outwitted, keep reminding yourself that you are grown-up and your toddler is not!

## hot dog and beans

**1 hot dog (2 oz),
    chopped coarsely**
**4 1/2 oz (1/2 cup) canned baked beans**
**1 medium tomato,
    chopped finely**
**1 mushroom, chopped finely**
**3 tablespoons chopped sweet red bell pepper**
**1/4 cup milk**

Combine all ingredients in small pan; bring to boil. Simmer, uncovered, until mixture thickens slightly. Serve with crusty bread or toast fingers.

MAKES 2 SERVINGS

**Storage** Covered, in refrigerator, up to 2 days
**Freeze** Suitable, in portion sizes

## beef 'n' veggie patties

**· 8 oz ground beef**
**1 small carrot,
    grated coarsely**
**1 small zucchini,
    grated coarsely**
**1 small potato,
    grated coarsely**
**1/2 small onion,
    chopped finely**
**1 1/2 tablespoons catsup**
**1 egg, beaten lightly**
**vegetable oil, for frying**

Using hand, combine beef, carrot, zucchini, potato, onion, catsup and egg in large bowl; shape rounded tablespoons of mixture into patties. Heat oil in medium pan; fry patties, in batches, until browned both sides and cooked through. Drain patties on paper towels; serve with noodles or rice, if desired.

MAKES ABOUT 20

**Storage** Uncooked mixture can be kept, covered, in refrigerator up to a day ahead
**Freeze** Suitable, uncooked, in individual portions

☺ TIP  This mixture also makes a tasty meat loaf; press in an oiled 3" x 10" loaf pan and bake at 350°F about 45 minutes or until firm and cooked through.

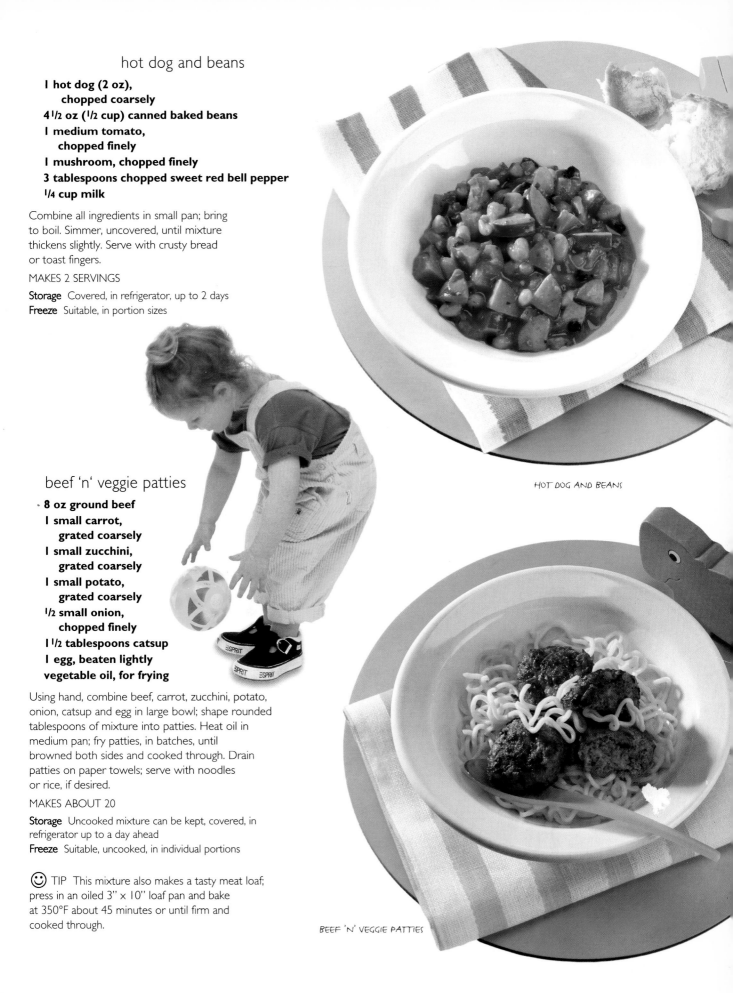

HOT DOG AND BEANS

BEEF 'N' VEGGIE PATTIES

## fish croquettes

**1 medium potato**
**4 oz (¹/₂ cup) canned salmon, drained**
**1 egg, beaten lightly**
**3 tablespoons finely grated carrot**
**3 tablespoons finely grated zucchini**
**3 tablespoons finely grated cheddar cheese**
**3 tablespoons all-purpose flour**
**2 teaspoons olive oil**

Boil, steam or microwave potato until tender; drain. Mash in small bowl; allow to cool. Meanwhile, remove and discard bones from salmon; combine salmon, egg, carrot, zucchini and cheese with potato. Using heaped tablespoons of mixture, shape into croquettes. Roll in flour, shake off excess. Heat oil in small non-stick pan; cook croquettes, in batches, until browned all over. Drain on paper towels; serve with lemon and tomato wedges and crustless bread.

MAKES 2 SERVINGS

**Storage** Uncooked mixture can be kept, covered, in refrigerator up to a day
**Freeze** Suitable, uncooked, in individual portions

☺ TIP  You can substitute canned tuna or steamed flaked fish fillet (be sure to remove any bones) for the salmon.

FISH CROQUETTES

## pizza fingers

**6" x 8" piece focaccia**
**²/₃ cup bottled tomato pasta sauce**
**1 medium tomato, halved, sliced**
**1 small sweet red bell pepper, chopped finely**
**2 oz (about ¹/₃ cup) mushrooms, sliced thinly**
**¹/₂ cup chopped ham**
**¹/₂ cup drained pineapple pieces**
**1 cup coarsely grated cheddar cheese**
**1 cup grated mozzarella cheese**

Split bread in half horizontally. Place bread, split-side up, on greased baking sheets; spread with sauce. Top with remaining ingredients; bake at 350°F about 15 minutes or until browned lightly. Cut into fingers to serve.

MAKES 2 TO 4 SERVINGS

*Must be made just before serving*

☺ TIP  You can also use cooked ground beef or other cooked chopped meat as part of the topping, if you desire. English muffins or a French bread loaf, halved through the center, can be used for the pizza base.

PIZZA FINGERS

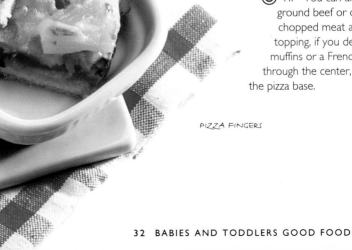

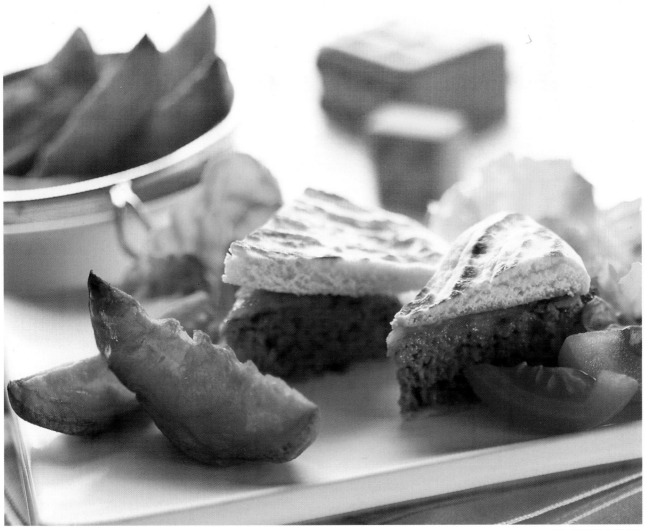

HAMBURGER WEDGES

## hamburger wedges

**8 oz ground beef**
**1/2 cup fresh breadcrumbs**
**1 egg, beaten lightly**
**3 tablespoons fruit chutney**
**1 1/2 tablespoons finely chopped fresh parsley**
**2 teaspoons olive oil**
**2 cheese slices**
**2 pieces pocket pita bread**
**3 tablespoons catsup**

Combine ground beef, breadcrumbs, egg, chutney and parsley in medium bowl; shape into 2 patties. Heat oil in medium pan; cook patties until browned both sides and cooked through. Place cheese on top of patties during last 5 minutes of cooking. Split pita in half, spread each bottom half with catsup; top with patties and remaining pita. Cut into wedges, serve with salad and crisp potato wedges.

MAKES 2 TO 4 SERVINGS

**Storage** Uncooked mixture can be kept, covered, in refrigerator up to a day
**Freeze** Suitable, uncooked, in individual portions

☺ TIP To prepare potato wedges, scrub 4 small potatoes; dry with paper towels, cut into wedges. Place wedges on greased baking tray, brush all over with olive oil. Bake, uncovered, at 450°F about 45 minutes or until browned.

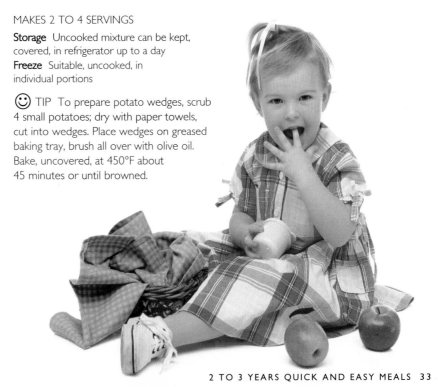

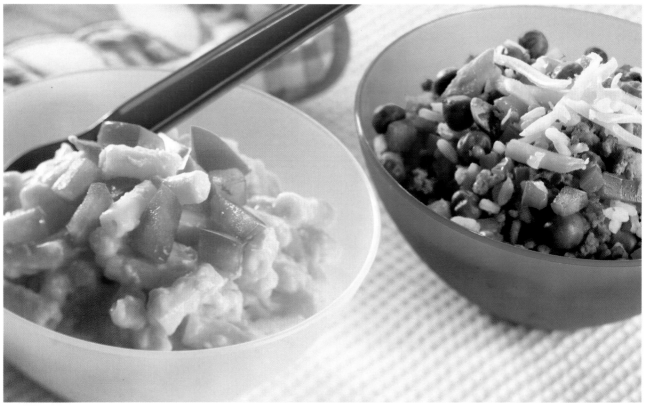

MACARONI CHEESE (LEFT) WITH BEEF AND VEGETABLE RICE

## macaroni cheese

*We used 1/2 cup uncooked short macaroni, but you can use elbow macaroni or even small pasta shells, if you wish.*

**2 tablespoons butter**
**1 1/2 tablespoons all-purpose flour**
**1 cup milk**
**1/2 cup coarsely grated cheddar cheese**
**1 1/3 cups cooked macaroni**

Heat butter in small pan, add flour; cook, stirring, until mixture thickens and bubbles. Gradually stir in milk; stir until mixture boils and thickens. Add cheese and macaroni; stir over heat until cheese melts and mixture is heated through. Top with chopped tomato, if desired.

MAKES 1 SERVING

**Storage** Covered, in refrigerator, up to 2 days

☺ TIP Place macaroni mixture in small oiled ovenproof dish; top with small amounts of finely chopped crisped bacon, chopped tomato, extra grated cheddar cheese and fresh breadcrumbs. Bake at 350°F about 10 minutes or until browned lightly.

## beef and vegetable rice

*About 1/8 cup of uncooked short grain rice makes the 1/2 cup cooked rice needed for this recipe.*

**2 teaspoons olive oil**
**2 oz ground beef**
**1 medium plum tomato, chopped finely**
**1 mushroom, chopped finely**
**1/4 cup frozen peas**
**1/2 cup cooked short grain rice**
**1/4 cup coarsely grated cheddar cheese**

Heat oil; cook ground beef, stirring, until browned. Add tomato, mushroom and peas; cook, stirring, until vegetables soften. Stir in rice; sprinkle with cheese.

MAKES 1 SERVING

**Storage** Covered, in refrigerator, up to 2 days
**Freeze** Suitable, in individual portions

☺ TIP Try adapting this recipe to make fried rice. Simply cook small amounts of finely chopped ham, green onions and drained canned corn kernels in medium pan; stir in cooked rice with a little soy sauce. You can also mix leftover vegetables or casseroles with cooked rice for a toddler's meal.

## fish 'n' chips

**1/4 cup all-purpose flour**
**1 1/2 tablespoons milk**
**3 tablespoons water**
**1 medium potato**
**vegetable oil, for deep frying**
**4 oz boneless white fish fillet**

Place flour in small bowl, gradually whisk in combined milk and water; cover, let stand 10 minutes. Cut potatoes into 3/8-inch slices; cut slices into 3/8-inch strips. Rinse potato strips under cold water, drain; dry with paper towels. Deep-fry potato strips in hot oil until browned lightly; drain on paper towels. Meanwhile, remove and discard any skin or bones from fish; cut fish into bite-size pieces. Dip fish in batter, drain off excess. Deep-fry fish, in batches, until browned and cooked through; drain on paper towels. Serve with mayonnaise for dipping, and if desired, with salad and crusty bread.

MAKES 1 SERVING

*Best made just before serving*

*difficult though it sometimes may be* try not to elevate sweet food to treat or reward status. It is very tempting to say, "If you eat this enormous and unappetizing plate of boiled spinach, then you can have this wonderfully sweet pudding." Look at it from the child's point of view: you are clearly indicating that the pudding is much more desirable than the veggies. What two-year-old is not going to hold out for the sweet stuff? She clamps her lips at the spinach, you refuse to serve the pudding and the battle is on! The solution? Serve a nutritious, low sugar dessert and if she wants to eat it first occasionally, the world will not come to a crashing halt.

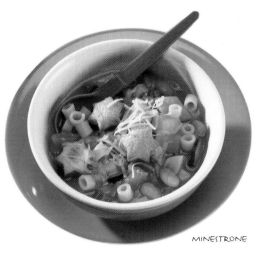

MINESTRONE

## minestrone

*This soup can be pureed for younger babies.*

1 1/2 **tablespoons olive oil**
1 **small onion,
     chopped finely**
1 **slice bacon, chopped finely**
1 **trimmed celery stalk,
     chopped finely**
1 **medium carrot,
     chopped finely**
1 **medium potato,
     chopped finely**
1 **medium zucchini,
     chopped finely**
14 1/2 **oz can tomatoes**
1 **cup canned mixed beans,
     drained**
1 **cup water**
1/2 **cup short tubular pasta**
1/4 **cup coarsely grated cheddar
     cheese**

Heat oil in large pan; cook onion and bacon, stirring, until onion is soft. Add celery, carrot, potato and zucchini; cook, stirring, until vegetables are just soft. Stir in undrained crushed tomatoes, beans, water and pasta; simmer, covered, 20 minutes or until vegetables and pasta are tender. Serve topped with cheese and homemade croutons, if desired.

MAKES 4 TO 6 SERVINGS

**Storage** Covered, in refrigerator, up to 2 days
**Freeze** Suitable, in individual portions

☺ TIP Toddlers love to be involved with their food: allow children to add their own cheese and croutons to the minestrone. Make croutons the quick and easy way by simply cutting toast into small cubes. Make more traditional croutons by baking crustless bread shapes at 350°F about 10 minutes, or by frying them in equal amounts of butter and oil until browned lightly; drain on paper towels.

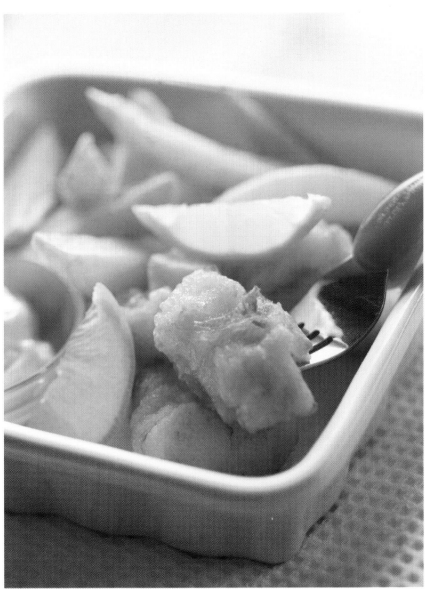

FISH 'N' CHIPS

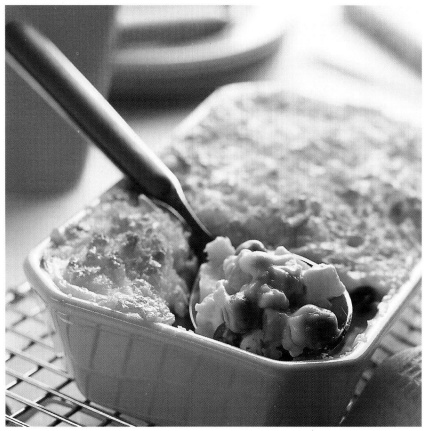

LEFTOVER ROAST DINNER CASSEROLE

## veggie pies with rice crusts

*You will need 2/3 cup uncooked short grain rice for the pie crusts.*

**1 1/2 cups cooked short grain rice**
**3 tablespoons finely grated parmesan cheese**
**1 egg yolk**

FILLING
**1 1/2 tablespoons butter**
**1/4 cup (2 oz) button mushrooms, chopped finely**
**1 small zucchini, grated coarsely**
**1/2 small tomato, chopped finely**
**1/2 cup ricotta cheese**
**1 egg yolk**

Oil deep 12-cup muffin tin or tart pan. Combine rice, cheese and egg yolk in small bowl; using wet hand, press 1 1/2 tablespoons of mixture over bottom of each cup in prepared pan. Spoon filling into rice shells; bake at 350°F about 25 minutes until filling is set and rice crusts browned lightly.

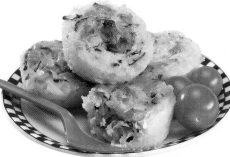

VEGGIE PIES WITH RICE CRUSTS

## leftover roast dinner casserole

**2 tablespoons butter**
**1 1/2 tablespoons all-purpose flour**
**1 cup milk**
**1 cup chopped cooked meat**
**1 cup chopped cooked vegetables**
**1/4 cup fresh breadcrumbs**
**1/2 cup coarsely grated cheddar cheese**

Heat butter in small pan, add flour; cook, stirring, until mixture thickens and bubbles. Gradually stir in milk; stir until mixture boils and thickens. Place combined meat and vegetables in shallow oiled 2-cup ovenproof dish; pour sauce over the top. Sprinkle with combined breadcrumbs and cheese; bake, uncovered, at 350°F about 20 minutes or until heated through and browned on top.

MAKES 2 TO 3 SERVINGS

*Best made just before serving*

## easy as pie

Place leftover seasoned ground meat, bolognese sauce, or a mild meat or vegetable curry in small greased ovenproof dishes; top with rounds of unfrozen prepackaged puff pastry. Brush with milk; pierce tops to create vents. Bake at 450°F about 10 minutes or until heated through and browned on top.

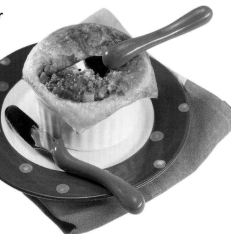

SEASONED GROUND MEAT TOPPED WITH PUFF PASTRY

**Filling** Heat butter in small pan; cook mushrooms, zucchini and tomato, stirring, until vegetables are soft. Remove from heat; stir in ricotta and egg yolk.

MAKES 12

**Storage** Covered, in refrigerator, up to 2 days
**Freeze** Suitable, in individual portions

# spreads for breads

Bread is one of life's great staples and the variety available these days
is nothing short of extraordinary. So, there is no excuse for white bread
boredom. As well as your usual loaf, let your toddler try wholegrain, rye, fruit
bread, French bread sticks, English muffins, bagels, soft tortilla, cracker or pita
bread and focaccia, to name but a few!

All of these breads can be topped or filled with any number of fillings that
your child enjoys – the combinations below are only the tip of the iceberg.
Remember too that this is a great way to disguise the vegetables and salads
that many toddlers try to avoid as their tastebuds become more selective.

## FILLINGS AND TOPPINGS
cheese slices with tomato
mashed avocado and sprouts
bologna, salami or any cold meat
cottage cheese and golden raisins with honey
tuna, celery and mayonnaise
banana with peanut butter and honey
peanut butter with finely grated carrot and golden raisins
anchovy paste

## GRILLED TOPPINGS
ham, pineapple and cheese
baked beans and cheese
sweet corn or corn kernels
  with finely grated cheddar cheese
sardines and catsup
cinnamon and sugar

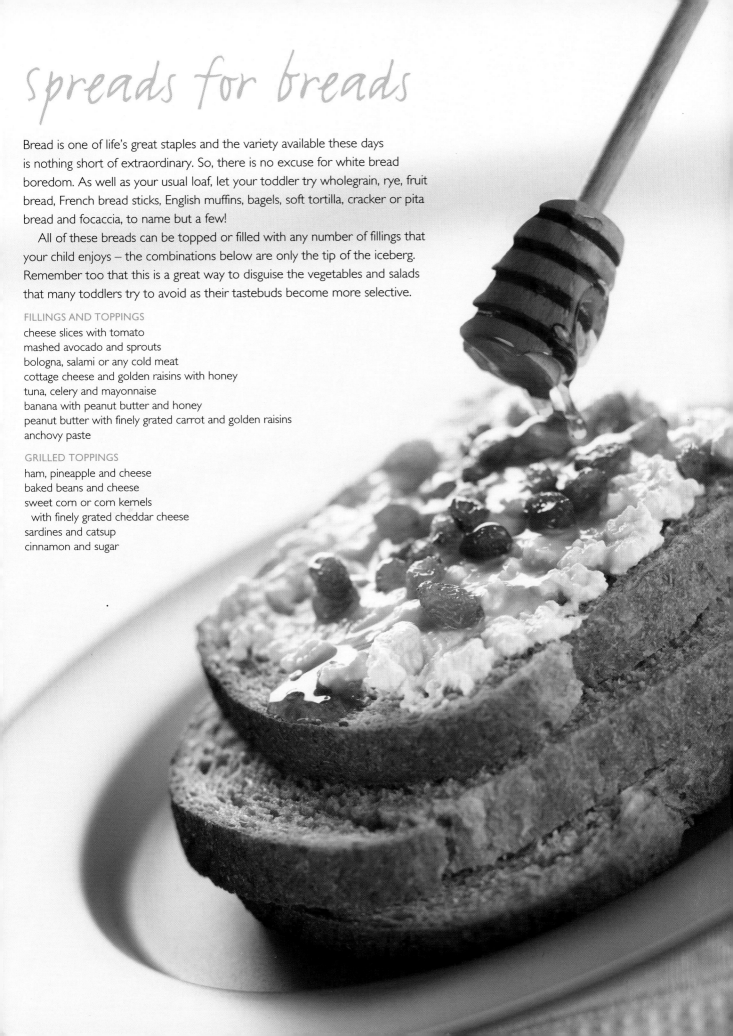

# The good egg

## bacon and vegetable omelette

**2 teaspoons butter**
**¹/₂ slice bacon, chopped**
**I egg, beaten lightly**
**I teaspoon milk or water**
**¹/₄ cup chopped**
    **cooked chicken**
**I ¹/₂ tablespoons canned corn**
    **kernels**
**I ¹/₂ tablespoons frozen peas,**
    **thawed, cooked**
**¹/₄ cup coarsely grated**
    **cheddar cheese**

Heat butter in small non-stick pan; cook bacon, stirring, until crisp. Pour combined egg and milk into pan; cook, tilting pan, over medium heat until mixture starts to set. Sprinkle remaining ingredients over omelette, fold in half; cook, uncovered, about I minute or until heated through. When almost set, sprinkle with cheese, fold in half.

Serve with chopped tomato, lettuce and bread triangles, if desired.

MAKES I SERVING

*Best made just before serving*

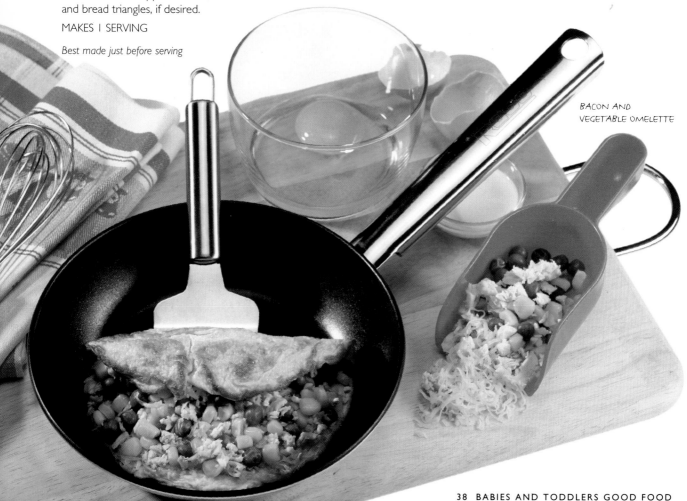

FRENCH TOAST

BACON AND VEGETABLE OMELETTE

## French toast

**2 slices bread**
**1 egg**
**1 ¹/₂ tablespoons milk**
**1 ¹/₂ tablespoons butter**

Remove crust from bread; cut each slice into 4 triangles. Whisk egg and milk in small bowl. Heat butter in medium pan; dip triangles, one at a time, in egg mixture, cook until browned both sides. Serve drizzled with maple syrup, if desired.

MAKES 1 SERVING

*Best made just before serving*

## egg florentine

**1 ¹/₂ tablespoons butter**
**2 teaspoons all-purpose flour**
**¹/₂ cup milk**
**¹/₄ cup coarsely grated cheddar cheese**
**2 oz (¹/₂ cup) frozen spinach, thawed**
**1 egg**
**1 ¹/₂ tablespoons grated cheddar cheese, extra**

Heat butter in small pan, add flour; cook, stirring, until mixture thickens and bubbles. Gradually stir in milk; stir until mixture boils and thickens, stir in cheese. Using hand, squeeze spinach to extract as much liquid as possible; place spinach in oiled ¹/₂-cup ovenproof dish. Press hollow in spinach with back of spoon; break egg over spinach, spoon sauce over spinach, sprinkle with extra cheese. Bake, uncovered, at 350°F about 10 minutes or until egg is set.

MAKES 1 SERVING

*Best made just before serving*

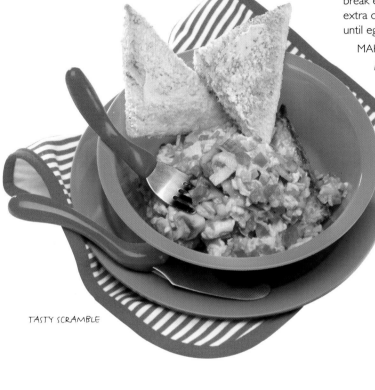

TASTY SCRAMBLE

## tasty scramble

**1 ¹/₂ tablespoons butter**
**2 oz (¹/₂ cup) lean ham, chopped finely**
**2 small button mushrooms, chopped finely**
**1 ¹/₂ tablespoons finely chopped tomato**
**1 egg, beaten lightly**
**1 ¹/₂ tablespoons milk**
**3 tablespoons coarsely grated cheddar cheese**

Heat butter in small pan; cook ham and mushrooms, stirring, until ham is browned. Stir in tomato and combined egg and milk; cook over low heat, stirring, until mixture starts to set. Stir in cheese; cook until mixture sets. Serve with buttered toast triangles.

MAKES 1 SERVING

*Best made just before serving*

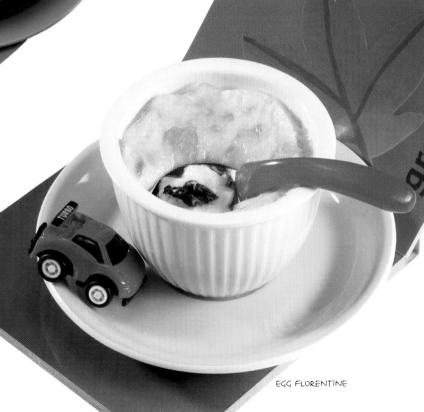

EGG FLORENTINE

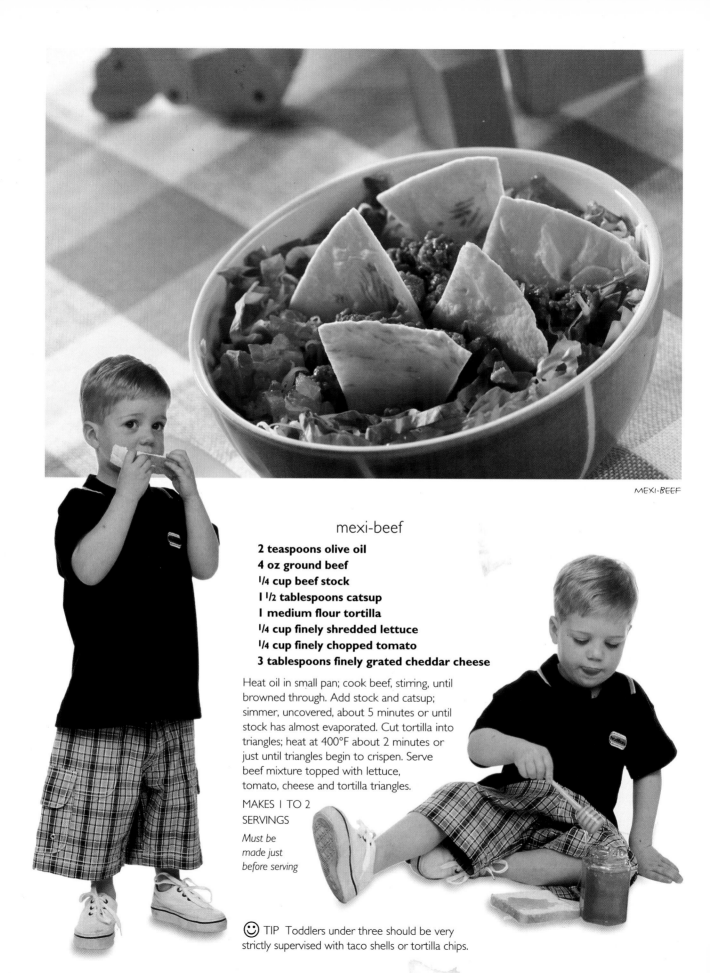

*MEXI-BEEF*

## mexi-beef

**2 teaspoons olive oil**
**4 oz ground beef**
**1/4 cup beef stock**
**1 1/2 tablespoons catsup**
**1 medium flour tortilla**
**1/4 cup finely shredded lettuce**
**1/4 cup finely chopped tomato**
**3 tablespoons finely grated cheddar cheese**

Heat oil in small pan; cook beef, stirring, until browned through. Add stock and catsup; simmer, uncovered, about 5 minutes or until stock has almost evaporated. Cut tortilla into triangles; heat at 400°F about 2 minutes or just until triangles begin to crispen. Serve beef mixture topped with lettuce, tomato, cheese and tortilla triangles.

MAKES 1 TO 2 SERVINGS

*Must be made just before serving*

☺ TIP Toddlers under three should be very strictly supervised with taco shells or tortilla chips.

# when is a sandwich not a sandwich?

Grilled sandwiches are the answer to a busy mother's prayer. They are quick, nourishing, easy to handle and different enough to persuade a fussy eater to take a bite.

Cheese is always the most requested filling in a grilled sandwich but it is easy to be more adventurous – within their crunchy sealed edges, these sandwiches can often provide a completely nutritious meal that your child will gladly eat in preference to a sit-down dinner.

**To make a grilled sandwich** Butter two slices of bread. Place your selected filling on the *unbuttered* side of one slice and top with remaining bread, buttered-side out. Place sandwich in a preheated electric sandwich maker. Cook until browned; cool 10 minutes before serving as **filling will be very hot.** Serve with salad (optimistic perhaps, but always worth a try).

### THE SUNDAY ROAST
Leftover roast, vegetables and gravy – remember to chop all solid ingredients into bite-size pieces

### CHICKEN FANTASTIQUE
Chopped cooked chicken with finely grated carrot, chopped avocado, mayonnaise

### HAWAIIAN WAVES
Lean ham, drained crushed pineapple, creamed corn

### ITALIAN GRILLED SANDWICH
Seasoned ground beef and grated parmesan cheese

### SALMON SUPREME
Canned flaked red salmon, chopped avocado, chopped tomato, cream cheese

### NUTTY SURPRISE
Chocolate hazelnut spread, dried apricots, ricotta cheese

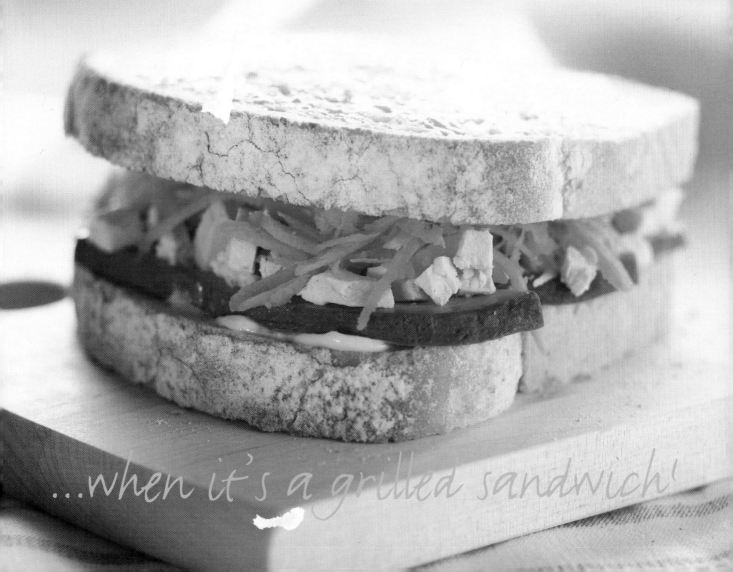

...when it's a grilled sandwich

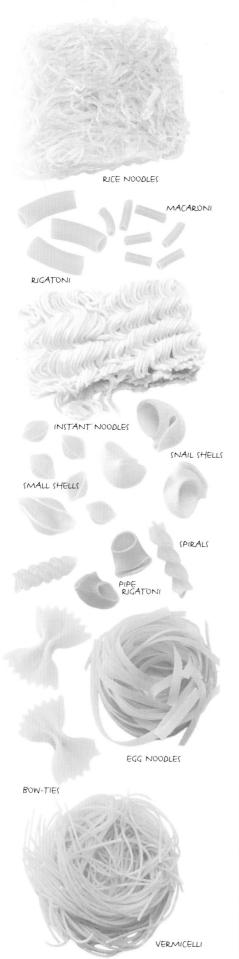

RICE NOODLES

MACARONI

RIGATONI

INSTANT NOODLES

SMALL SHELLS

SNAIL SHELLS

SPIRALS

PIPE RIGATONI

EGG NOODLES

BOW-TIES

VERMICELLI

## chicken 'n' noodles

**1/2 packet (3 oz) instant noodles
    chicken-flavored (ramen)**
**1 cup boiling water**
**1 teaspoon vegetable oil**
**1 green onion, chopped**
**1 boneless chicken thigh (4 oz),
    sliced thinly**
**3 snow peas, sliced thinly**
**3 green beans, sliced thinly**
**1/4 cup sliced carrot**
**1/4 cup sliced zucchini**
**2 teaspoons soy sauce**

Combine noodles and boiling water in
small bowl; let stand 2 minutes. Stir in half
of the seasoning packet; drain over small
bowl, reserve 1/4 cup of the liquid. Heat
oil in wok or medium pan; stir-fry chicken
until browned and cooked through.
Remove chicken from wok; cover to
keep warm. Add vegetables to wok; stir-
fry about 3 minutes or until just tender.
Return chicken to wok with noodles,
reserved liquid and soy sauce; stir-fry
until heated through.

MAKES 1 SERVING

*Best made just before serving*

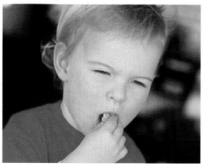

## spring rolls

**2 teaspoons olive oil**
**3 green onions, chopped finely**
**1 small carrot, finely grated**
**1 small zucchini,
    coarsely grated**
**3/4 cup finely
    shredded cabbage**
**1/2 cup bean sprouts**
**4 oz ground lamb**
**3/4 cup coarsely grated
    cheddar cheese**
**12 sheets filo pastry**
**1/4 cup olive oil, extra**

Heat oil in wok or medium pan; stir-fry
onion, carrot, zucchini, cabbage and
sprouts 2 minutes. Add lamb, stir-fry until
browned and cooked through. Remove
from heat, stir in cheese; cool. Cover filo
with slightly damp cloth until ready to use
to prevent its drying out. Remove 1 sheet
filo; brush with extra oil, fold in half
lengthwise then in half crosswise. Fold
again to form a 4" x 5" rectangle; brush
with more oil. Place 1 1/2 heaped
tablespoons of the filling mixture on each
square; roll, folding in sides as you go.
Brush lightly with oil; place on oiled
baking sheet. Repeat with remaining filo
and filling mixture. Bake at 400°F about
15 minutes or until browned. Serve
with sweet and sour or tomato sauce,
if desired.

MAKES 12

**Storage** Uncooked mixture can be kept,
covered, in refrigerator several hours ahead
**Freeze** Suitable, uncooked, individually

☺ TIP  Ground chicken can be
substituted for lamb.

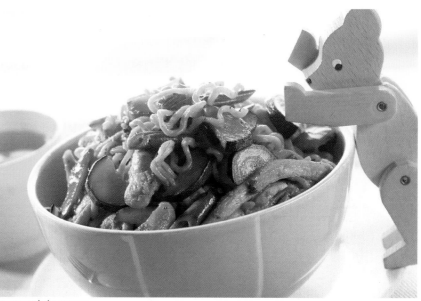

CHICKEN 'N' NOODLES

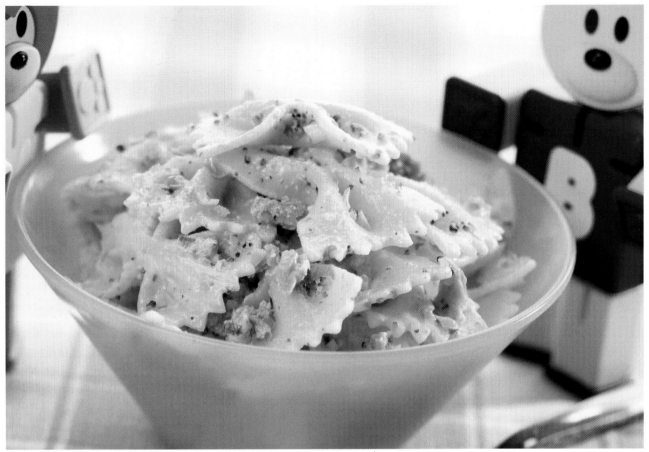

SALMON AND BROCCOLI PASTA

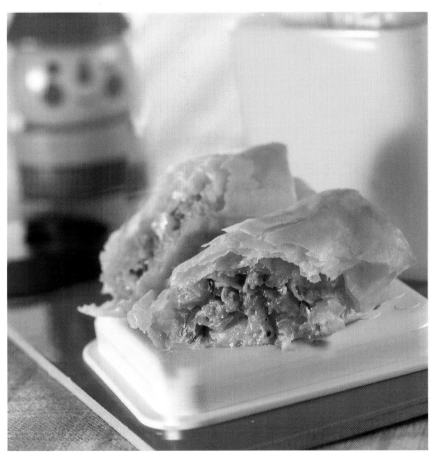

SPRING ROLLS

## salmon and broccoli pasta

*We used bow-tie pasta (farfelle) but you can use any sort of short pasta in this recipe.*

**2 teaspoons butter**
**1 green onion, chopped finely**
**3 tablespoons finely**
**    chopped broccoli**
**1 1/2 tablespoons water**
**1 1/2 tablespoons spreadable**
**    cream cheese**
**1 1/2 tablespoons drained canned**
**    red salmon**
**1/2 cup pasta**

Heat butter in small pan; cook onion, broccoli and water, stirring, until broccoli is tender. Add cream cheese; cook, stirring, until melted. Stir in salmon. Meanwhile, cook pasta in medium pan of boiling water, uncovered, until just tender; drain. Gently toss pasta in small bowl with salmon mixture.

MAKES 1 SERVING
*Best made just before serving.*

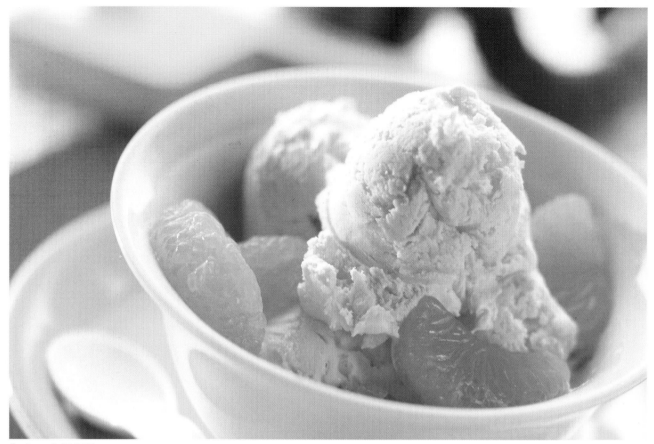

QUICK-MIX ICE CREAM

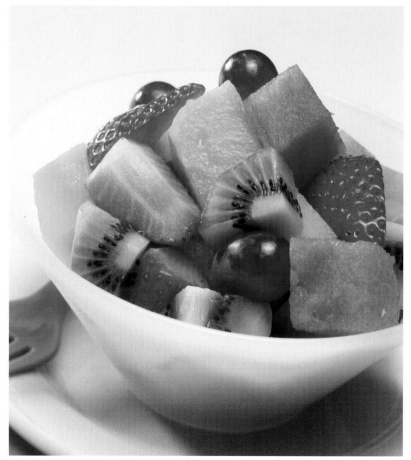

FRUIT SALAD

## quick-mix ice cream

**2 1/2 cups cream**
**14 oz can condensed milk**
**1 teaspoon vanilla extract**

Beat cream in small bowl with electric mixer until soft peaks form; gently fold in milk and vanilla. Pour mixture into deep 8-inch square cake pan, cover with foil; freeze overnight or until firm.

MAKES 8 SERVINGS

☺ TIP  Fold through grated chocolate or pureed fruit before freezing ice cream.

## frozen yogurt

Puree 1/2 cup chopped fresh fruit of your choice; fold into 7 ounces vanilla yogurt in small bowl. Pour into an ice tray; freeze overnight or until firm.

## fruit salad

Chop up a combination of your favorite seasonal fruits to make an appealing "finger food" for your child. Serve with custard or yogurt, if desired.

☺ TIP  Choose seedless grapes, or halve seeded grapes and remove seeds for toddlers under the age of four.

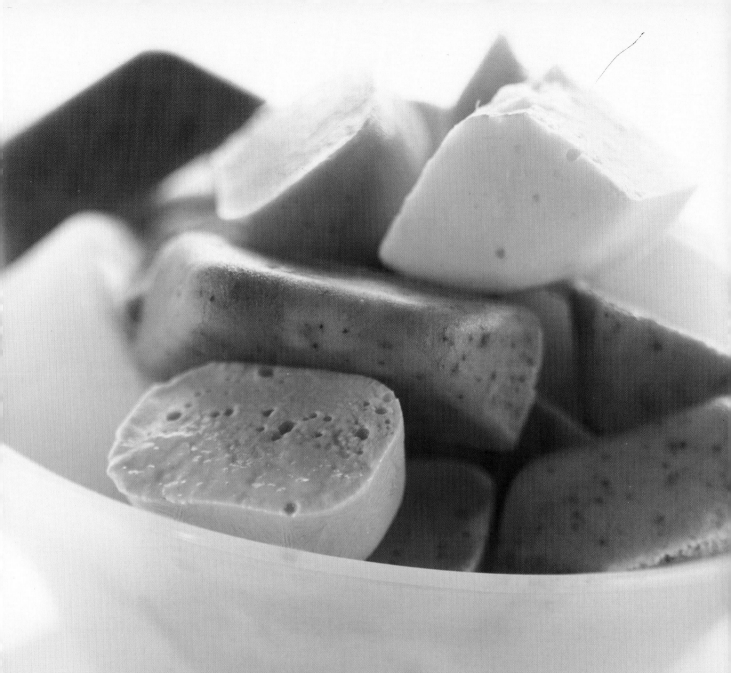

frozen yogurt. yum! yum!

# snacking and finger food

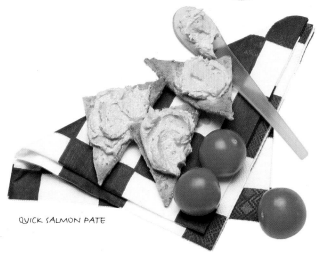

QUICK SALMON PATE

These recipes are designed to add variety to the range of foods your toddler is now eating. Although we call them snacks, any of them could form the basis of a meal, and all of them pass the ultimate toddler test: they can be picked up and eaten with the fingers! They are ideal for that time of the afternoon when lunch seems a long time ago, dinner is still some way off and food of some sort is definitely called for – after all, just *being* 2 or 3 years old uses the most amazing amount of energy! A nutritious snack is also useful if your toddler is the "grazing" variety, who wants small amounts of food fairly frequently.

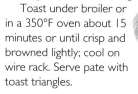

## quick salmon pate

*This is a versatile recipe: you can serve it on toast at breakfast, as a sandwich filling at lunch, or tossed through hot pasta for dinner.*

**4 oz (½ cup) canned red salmon, drained**
**2 oz (¼ cup) packaged cream cheese**
**¼ cup mayonnaise**
**2 teaspoons lemon juice**
**2 teaspoons chopped fresh parsley**
**3 tablespoons butter, softened**
**6 slices multi-grain bread**

Remove skin and bones from salmon; process salmon, cream cheese, mayonnaise, juice, parsley and butter until pureed. Remove crusts from bread and flatten with a rolling pin. Cut each bread slice into 4 triangles; place on baking sheet.

Toast under broiler or in a 350°F oven about 15 minutes or until crisp and browned lightly; cool on wire rack. Serve pate with toast triangles.

MAKES 1 CUP PATE

**Storage** Pate, covered, in refrigerator up to 2 days; Toasts, airtight container up to 1 week

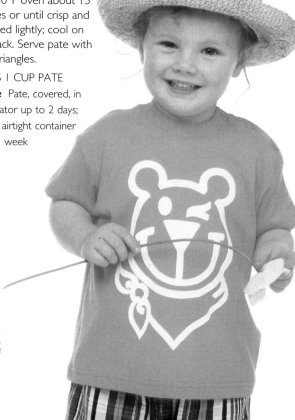

## popcorn

**1 1/2 tablespoons vegetable oil**
**1/4 cup popping corn**

Heat oil in large pan; pop popcorn, covered tightly, over medium heat, shaking occasionally, until popping stops. Remove from heat; pour into large serving bowl; cool before serving.

MAKES ABOUT 5 CUPS

**Storage** Airtight container, up to 2 days

☺ TIP Popcorn can also be prepared in a microwave oven. Place corn, without oil, in microwave-safe bowl; cover tightly with plastic wrap, cook on HIGH (100%) about 3 minutes or until popping stops.

**Do not serve to toddlers under 3 years of age**

## French onion dip

**2/3 cup sour cream**
**1 1/2 tablespoons French onion soup mix**

Combine ingredients in small bowl; serve with toddler's favorite raw or blanched vegetables.

MAKES 2/3 CUP

**Storage** Covered, in refrigerator, up to 2 days

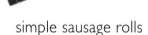
SAUSAGE ROLLS

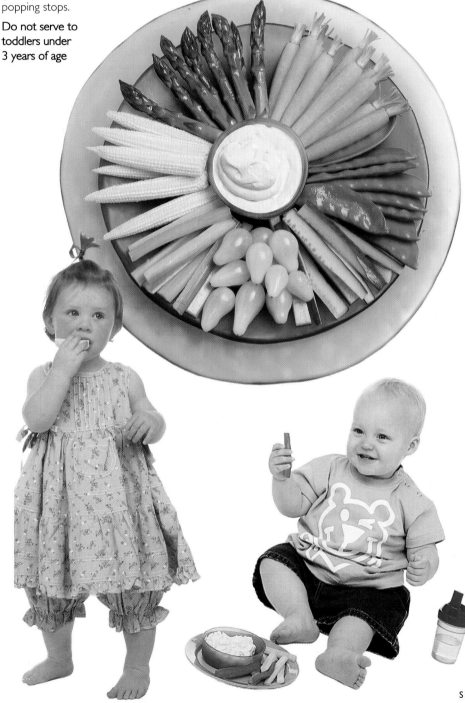
FRENCH ONION DIP WITH VEGETABLES

## simple sausage rolls

**1 sheet unfrozen prepackaged puff pastry**
**2 teaspoons milk**
**4 thin beef sausages (8 oz)**
**2 teaspoons fresh breadcrumbs**

Cut pastry in half; brush with half the milk. Place 2 sausages, end to end, along center of each pastry half; trim sausages to fit pastry. Roll pastry to enclose sausages; place, seam-side down, on greased baking sheet.

Brush with remaining milk, sprinkle with breadcrumbs. Bake at 400°F about 15 minutes or until pastry is browned lightly and sausages are cooked through. Cut each roll diagonally into 5 pieces. Serve with tomato sauce, if desired.

MAKES 10

**Storage** Covered, in refrigerator, up to 2 days
**Freeze** Uncooked sausage rolls suitable

POPCORN

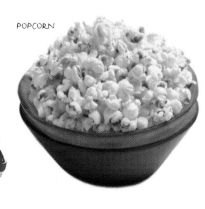

## basic scones

**2 1/2 cups self-rising flour**
**1 1/2 tablespoons superfine sugar**
**1/4 teaspoon salt**
**2 tablespoons butter**
**3/4 cup milk**
**1/2 cup water,**
   **approximately**

Grease 9-inch square layer cake pan.
Place flour, sugar and salt in medium
bowl; rub in butter with fingertips. Using a
knife, stir in milk and enough water to
make a soft, sticky dough.

Turn dough onto floured surface;
knead quickly and lightly until smooth.
Use hand to press dough out evenly to
3/4-inch thickness; cut into 2-inch rounds.

Gently knead scraps of dough together,
repeat pressing and cutting out of dough.
Place scones in prepared pan; bake at
500°F about 15 minutes or until scones
are browned and sound hollow when
tapped. Turn onto wire rack to cool. Serve
with jam and cream, if desired.

MAKES 16

**Freeze** Cooked or uncooked scones suitable

☺ **TIP** If you prefer crusty scones, cool
uncovered. To soften crust, wrap hot
scones in a kitchen towel.

## cheesy pumpkin and zucchini scones

**2 1/2 cups self-rising flour**
**1 1/2 tablespoons superfine sugar**
**1/4 teaspoon salt**
**2 tablespoons butter**
**1/4 cup finely grated pumpkin**
   **or winter squash**
**1/4 cup finely**
   **grated zucchini**
**1/4 cup finely grated**
   **cheddar cheese**
**3/4 cup milk**
**1/4 cup water,**
   **approximately**
**3 tablespoons finely grated**
   **parmesan cheese**

Grease 9-inch square layer cake pan.
Place flour, sugar and salt into bowl; rub
in butter with fingertips. Stir in pumpkin,
zucchini and cheddar cheese. Using a
knife, stir in milk and enough water to
make a soft, sticky dough.

Proceed as in Basic Scone recipe
above. Before baking scones, sprinkle
with parmesan cheese.

MAKES 16

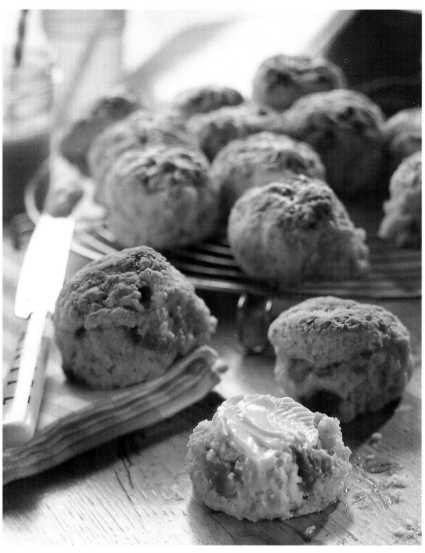

FROM BACK: CHEESY PUMPKIN AND ZUCCHINI SCONES AND APRICOT WHOLEWHEAT SCONES

## apricot wholewheat scones

**1/2 cup finely chopped**
   **dried apricots**
**1/2 cup boiling water**
**1 1/2 cups self-rising flour**
**1 cup wholewheat**
   **self-rising flour**
**1 1/2 tablespoons superfine sugar**
**1/4 teaspoon salt**
**2 tablespoons butter**
**3/4 cup milk,**
   **approximately**

Grease 9-inch square layer cake pan.
Place apricots in heatproof bowl, add
boiling water; let stand for 15 minutes.
Place flours, sugar and salt in large bowl;
rub in butter with fingertips. Using a knife,
stir in undrained apricot mixture and
enough milk to make a soft, sticky dough.

Proceed as in Basic Scone recipe
above.

MAKES 16

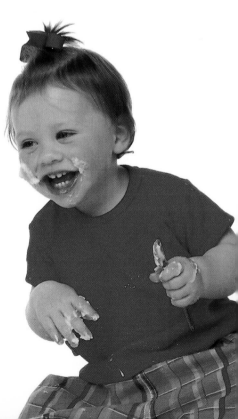

## chicken corn pouches

**5 oz ground chicken**
**3 tablespoons corn kernels**
**2 teaspoons light soy sauce**
**1 green onion, chopped finely**
**pinch five-spice powder**
**3 tablespoons canned finely**
**chopped water chestnuts**
**16 spring roll wrappers (5" x 5")**
**1 egg, beaten lightly**
**vegetable oil, for deep frying**

Combine chicken, corn, sauce, onion, spice and chestnuts in small bowl; mix well. Place rounded teaspoon of chicken mixture on center of each wrapper; brush around edge with egg, form into pouch shape, pinch to seal.

Deep-fry pouches in hot oil, in batches, until browned and cooked through. Drain on paper towels. Serve with plum sauce, if desired.

MAKES 16

*Best prepared on day of use; deep-fry just before serving*

**Freeze** Uncooked pouches suitable

## vegetable fritters

**¹/₃ cup cauliflower florets**
**¹/₃ cup broccoli florets**
**¹/₄ cup all-purpose flour**
**1 ¹/₂ tablespoons cornstarch**
**1 ¹/₂ tablespoons polenta**
**¹/₂ teaspoon powdered chicken**
**bouillon**
**1 egg white**
**¹/₄ cup water**
**¹/₂ small zucchini, sliced thickly**
**¹/₂ small orange sweet potato,**
**sliced thickly**
**vegetable oil, for deep-frying**

Boil, steam or microwave cauliflower and broccoli, separately, until just tender; drain. Place flours, polenta and salt in small bowl; stir in egg white and water, mix to smooth batter. Dip vegetables in batter to coat completely. Deep-fry vegetables in hot oil, in batches, until browned lightly and crisp. Drain on paper towels.

MAKES 2 SERVINGS

*Best made just before serving*

☺ TIP Poppadums, or traditional Indian crackers, are healthy snacks: cook, 1 at a time, in the microwave oven on HIGH (100%) about 50 seconds or until puffed and crisp. Serve alone or with dips to toddlers over 3 years of age.

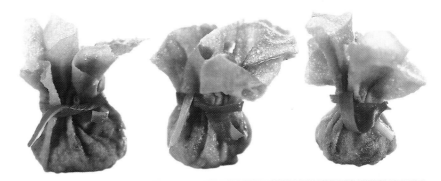

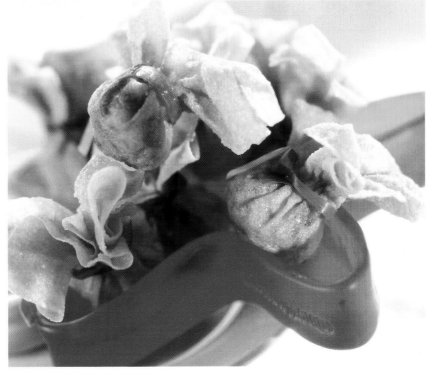

CHICKEN CORN POUCHES

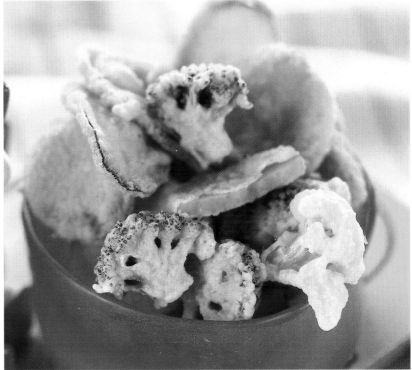

VEGETABLE FRITTERS

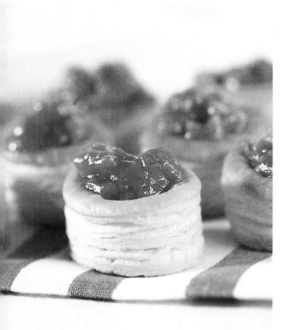

TOMATO TASTIES

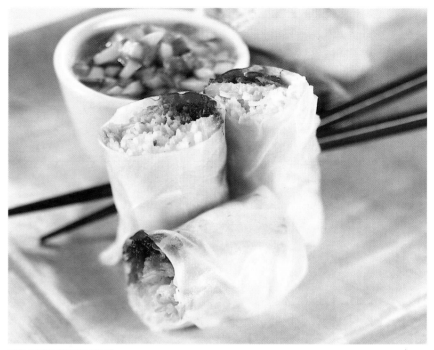

RICE-PAPER VEGGIE ROLLS

## tomato tasties

*Round or oval pastry shells made of puff or flaky pastry are available in supermarkets in packages of 12.*

**12 puff pastry shells
1 button mushroom, chopped finely
1/3 cup bottled tomato pasta sauce**

Place puff pastry shells on baking sheet; bake at 375°F 5 minutes.
Meanwhile, combine mushroom and sauce in small pan; cook, stirring, until hot. Fill shells just before serving; refrigerate or freeze remaining sauce for use in other snacks.

MAKES 12

**Storage** Sauce, covered, in refrigerator up to 4 days. Puff pastry shells, in airtight container, up to 1 week
**Freeze** Sauce and puff pastry shells suitable

## rice-paper veggie rolls

*We used bean thread noodles for this simple recipe which makes a healthy snack for children and adults alike.*

**1 oz bean thread noodles
2 teaspoons smooth peanut butter
2 teaspoons hot water**

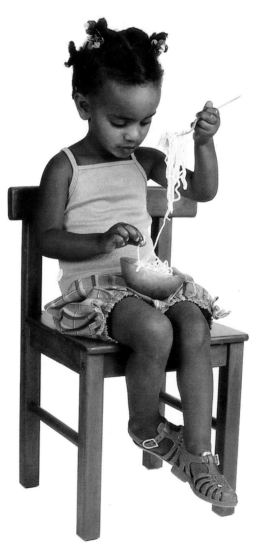

**4 sheets rice paper
1/4 small avocado, sliced thinly
1/2 small carrot, grated finely
3 tablespoons finely grated fresh beets
1 green onion, sliced finely**

DIPPING SAUCE
**3 tablespoons sugar
3 tablespoons water
1 1/2 tablespoons white vinegar
1/2 burpless cucumber, seeded, chopped finely**

Place bean threads in small heatproof bowl, cover with boiling water, let stand only until just tender; drain. Cut noodles into 1 1/2-inch lengths; combine in small bowl with peanut butter and the hot water. Place 1 sheet of rice paper in medium bowl of warm water until just softened; lift out carefully, place on board. Place layer of noodle mixture in center of rice paper; top with avocado, carrot, beets and onion. Roll to enclose, folding in ends.
Repeat with remaining rice paper sheets and filling ingredients. Serve with Dipping Sauce.

**Dipping Sauce** Combine sugar and water in small pan; stir over low heat, without boiling, until sugar dissolves. Simmer, uncovered, 2 minutes; stir in vinegar, cool. Stir in cucumber.

MAKES 4

*Best assembled just before serving*

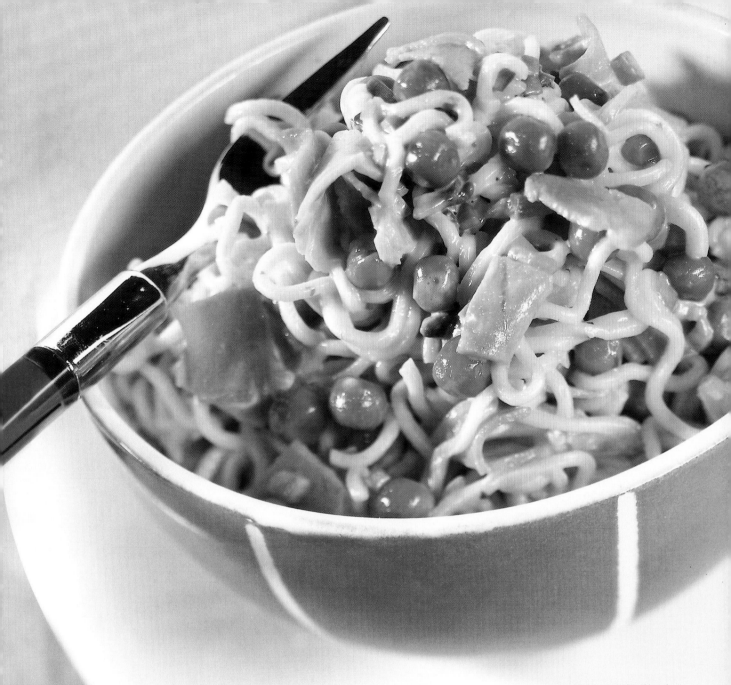

MUSHROOMS, PEAS, HAM AND
CREAM NOODLES

# using your noodle

Most small children adore instant noodles and from the cook's point of view they are a good idea as well, since they are ready in minutes, provide a satisfying serving of energy-giving carbohydrates, and can be combined with an infinite variety of ingredients to suit the taste and appetite of even the fussiest eater. Instant noodles can be purchased in a plain, unflavored form, but if you are using the sort that comes with a seasoning packet, be aware that this flavoring can taste very strong to a young palate and is often too salty. When preparing the noodles for a child, either discard the seasoning packet altogether, or only use a very small amount, then combine the noodles with the ingredients of your choice, or try one of the suggestions listed here:

• tuna, green onions and tomato  • mushrooms, peas, ham and a little cream
• chicken with creamed corn or corn kernels  • stir-fried mixed vegetables

## corn mini pancakes

**1 cup self-rising flour**
**3/4 cup milk**
**1 egg**
**1 1/2 tablespoons butter, melted**
**4 1/2 oz (1/2 cup) canned creamed
   corn**
**2 green onions, chopped finely**
**1/4 cup finely chopped
   sweet red bell pepper**
**1/4 cup grated cheddar cheese**

Place flour in medium bowl; gradually stir in combined milk, egg and butter, mix to a smooth batter. Stir in remaining ingredients. Drop by 1/4 cupsful of mixture, in batches, into heated oiled heavy-bottomed pan, cook until bubbles appear; turn mini pancakes, cook until brown. Serve with sour cream.

MAKES 8

**Storage** Covered, in refrigerator, up to 2 days
**Freeze** Suitable

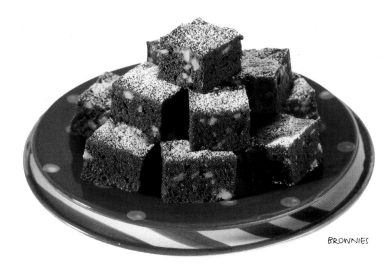

BROWNIES

## potato mini pancakes

**1 cup self-rising flour**
**3/4 cup milk**
**1 egg**
**1 1/2 tablespoons butter, melted**
**1 clove garlic, crushed**
**1 small onion,
   grated coarsely**
**1 small potato,
   grated coarsely**

Place flour in medium bowl; gradually stir in combined milk, egg and butter, mix to a smooth batter. Stir in remaining ingredients. Drop by 1/4 cupsful of mixture, in batches, into heated oiled heavy-bottomed pan, cook until bubbles appear; turn mini pancakes, cook until brown. Serve with sour cream.

MAKES 8

**Storage** Covered, in refrigerator, up to 2 days
**Freeze** Suitable

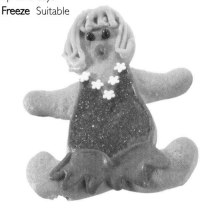

## brownies

**10 tablespoons butter**
**1 cup firmly packed
   brown sugar**
**2 eggs**
**1/2 cup all-purpose flour**
**1/2 cup cocoa**
**1/2 cup finely
   chopped pecans**

Grease deep 8-inch square cake pan, line bottom and sides with parchment paper. Beat butter and sugar in small bowl with electric mixer until light and fluffy. Add eggs, 1 at a time, beating until just combined between additions. Stir in sifted flour and cocoa, then nuts; spread mixture into prepared pan. Bake at 300°F about 30 minutes; cool in pan. Cut into small squares; dust with sifted powdered sugar, if desired.

**Storage** Airtight container, up to 4 days
**Freeze** Suitable

**Omit nuts if serving to toddlers under 5 years of age**

FROM BACK: POTATO MINI PANCAKES AND CORN MINI PANCAKES

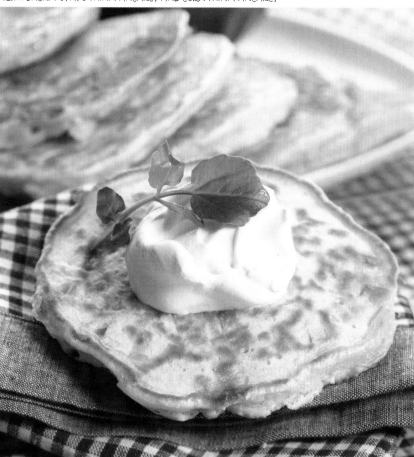

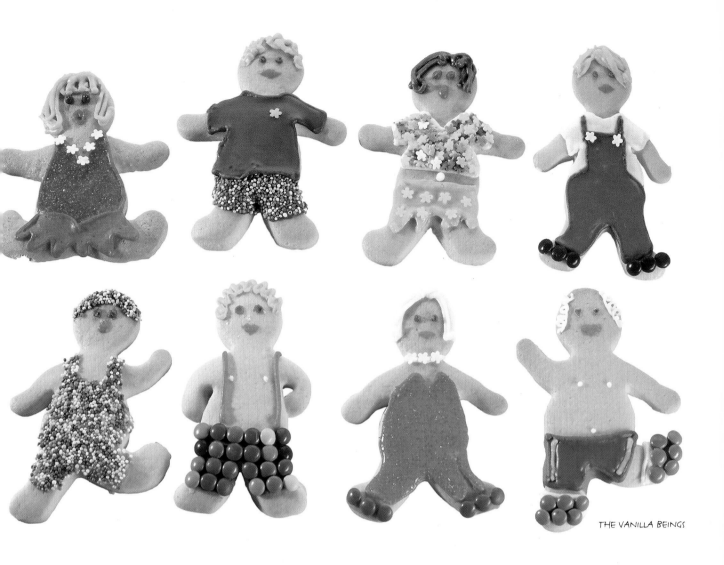

THE VANILLA BEINGS

# the vanilla beings

*Cutters of many shapes and sizes are available from kitchen shops and department stores. The number you get from one quantity of dough will depend on the size of cutters: we used a 4-inch gingerbread cutter here. You also need assorted food colorings, piping bags and sprinkles or cake decors to decorate these cookies.*

**1/2 cup butter**
**1 teaspoon vanilla extract**
**2/3 cup superfine sugar**
**2 eggs, beaten lightly**
**2 teaspoons milk**
**1 1/3 cups self-rising flour**
**1 cup all-purpose flour**

**ICING**
**2 egg whites**
**3 1/2 cups powdered sugar**

Beat butter, vanilla and sugar in medium bowl with electric mixer until smooth.

Add eggs, one at a time; beat until just combined. Stir in milk and flours; mix to a soft dough. Knead dough on floured surface until smooth, cover; refrigerate 30 minutes. Roll dough between sheets of waxed paper until 1/4-inch thick. Using 4-inch cutter, cut shapes from dough, re-rolling dough as necessary.

Place shapes, about 1 inch apart, on lightly greased cookie sheets; bake at 350°F about 10 minutes or until cookies are firm and browned lightly. Let stand 5 minutes; lift cookies onto wire racks and allow to cool.

**Icing** Beat egg whites in medium bowl with electric mixer until soft peaks form; gradually beat in powdered sugar. Divide among as many small bowls as you need for different colors; tint as desired with food colorings.

Spoon icing into piping bags fitted with plain tubes; decorate cooled cookies with icing and sprinkles or cake decors.

MAKES ABOUT 20

**Storage** Airtight container, up to 1 week
**Freeze** Unfrosted cookies suitable

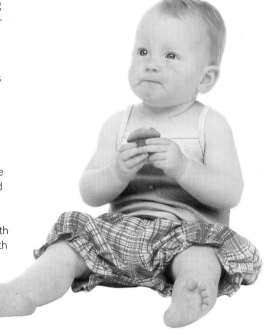

## popsicles

*For variety, try using other fruit juice flavors or soft drink.*

**¹/₂ cup natural yogurt**
**2 cups apple juice**
**1 cup black currant juice**

Place yogurt in large mixing bowl, gradually whisk in apple juice. Pour half the yogurt mixture into twelve ¹/₃-cup popsicle molds or paper cups; freeze until almost set. Insert a popsicle stick into center of popsicle; return to freezer until set. Pour black currant juice on top of frozen yogurt layer; freeze until firm. Top with remaining yogurt mixture; freeze until firm.

MAKES 12

☺ TIP  Vary the flavor and texture of these popsicles by using juice or syrup from canned fruit, diluted to taste.

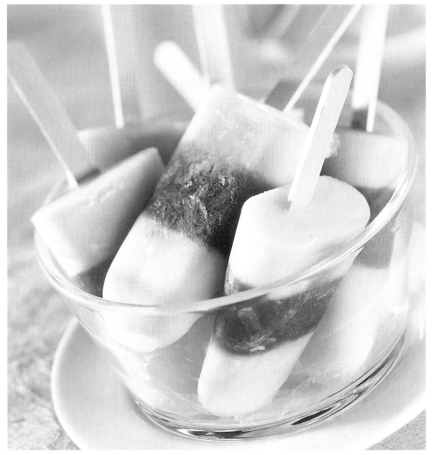

POPSICLES

QUICK APPLE TARTS

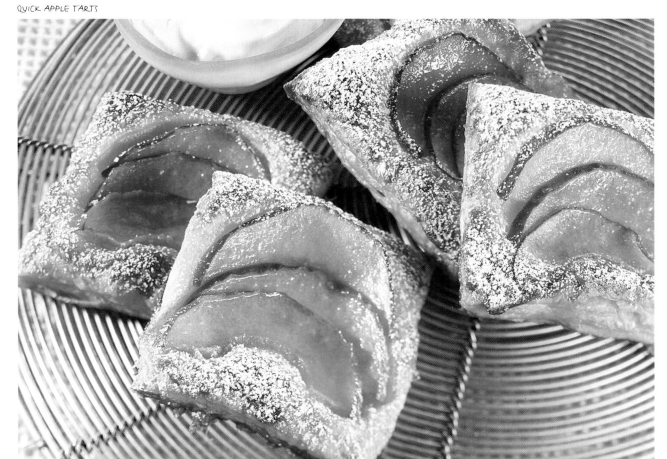

## goody bags

Prepare a bag of mixed treats – they are ideal for a snack pack to carry in your backpack and for your child when she is traveling in the stroller. Create your own selection or try one of the suggestions listed here:

- fruit sticks • apricot and coconut slice
- pretzels • small cracker shapes
- small cookies • golden raisins

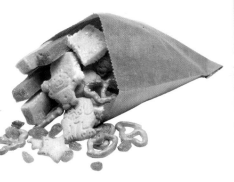

## smoothie

*We used fresh strawberries here but a banana or 1/2 cup of cantaloupe pieces also make a great smoothie.*

**1/2 cup milk**
**1/2 cup sliced strawberries**
**1/4 cup strawberry yogurt**

Blend all ingredients until smooth.

MAKES ABOUT 1 CUP

*Best made just before serving*

## quick apple tarts

**1 unfrozen puff pastry sheet**
**3 tablespoons butter, melted**
**1 medium apple, cored, sliced thinly**
**1 1/2 tablespoons brown sugar**
**1 1/2 tablespoons superfine sugar**
**1 1/2 tablespoons powdered sugar**

Cut pastry into 9 squares; place on greased baking sheet. Using half the butter, brush each square; divide apple slices among squares, brush with remaining butter. Sprinkle with brown and superfine sugars; bake at 450°F about 30 minutes or until puffed and browned lightly. Lift onto wire rack to cool; dust with powdered sugar before serving.

MAKES 9

**Storage** Covered, in refrigerator, up to 2 days
**Freeze** Uncooked tarts suitable

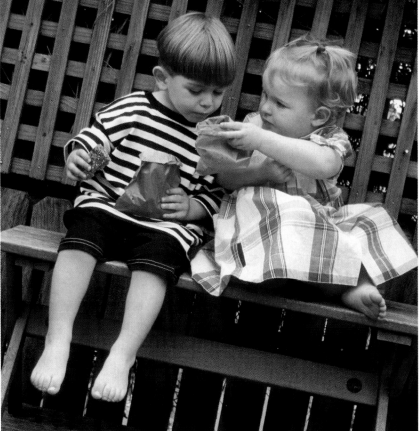

SMOOTHIE

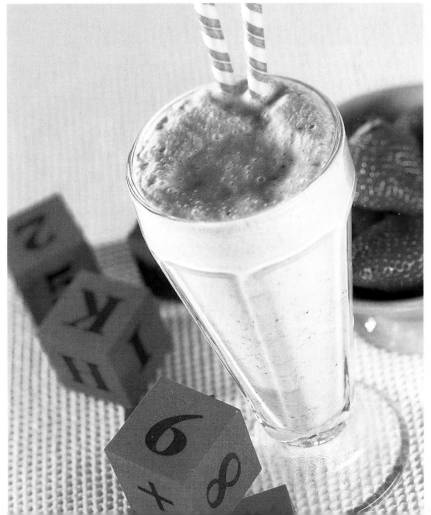

# portable food and lunchboxes

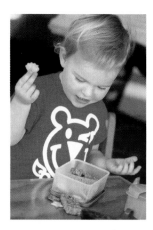

Aside from occasionally being a necessity, portable food is another excellent way of making a mealtime enjoyable for your toddler. Even if you only sit on a rug at the end of your yard, the idea of a picnic almost invariably appeals to a small child and presents a wonderful opportunity for involving her in the preparations and sense of adventure. For the difficult eater, too, taking a meal into different surroundings can defuse a stressful situation and, with any luck, create renewed interest in eating. And if it does neither of those things, at least you can enjoy the sunshine and rejoice that this is one meal you will not need to scrape from the walls!

### Eating outdoors

Whether you are in the garden or in the local park with the neighborhood mothers, choose food that is easy to pack and carry and, of course, easy to eat with the fingers. It is a good idea to invest in an inexpensive set of plastic containers of varying sizes, all with tight-fitting lids, as well as some unbreakable tumblers or plastic screw-top bottles, for drinks. And do not forget washcloths or tissues – the potential for mess remains fairly constant!

### Eating and travel

When considering a journey with small children, it is sensible to take along an insulated bag or small cooler, as food can deteriorate quickly in a hot car. Pack lots of small snack-type foods and plenty of fluids – children become irritable when constrained for any length of time and snacking is a sure way to divert their attention and keep up flagging energy levels. You should take care, however, when traveling alone with small toddlers, to give them only food that they cannot choke on – if you are in any doubt, stop the car so that you can supervise the snack.

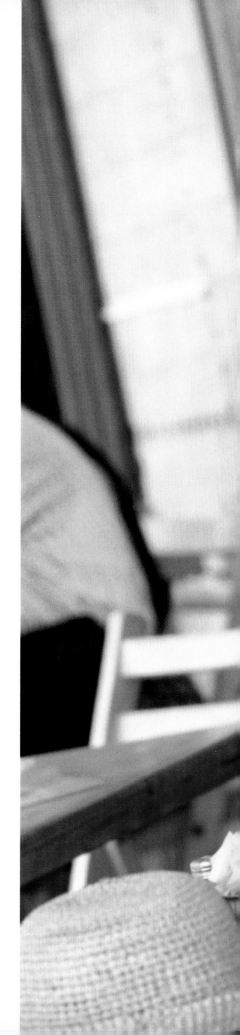

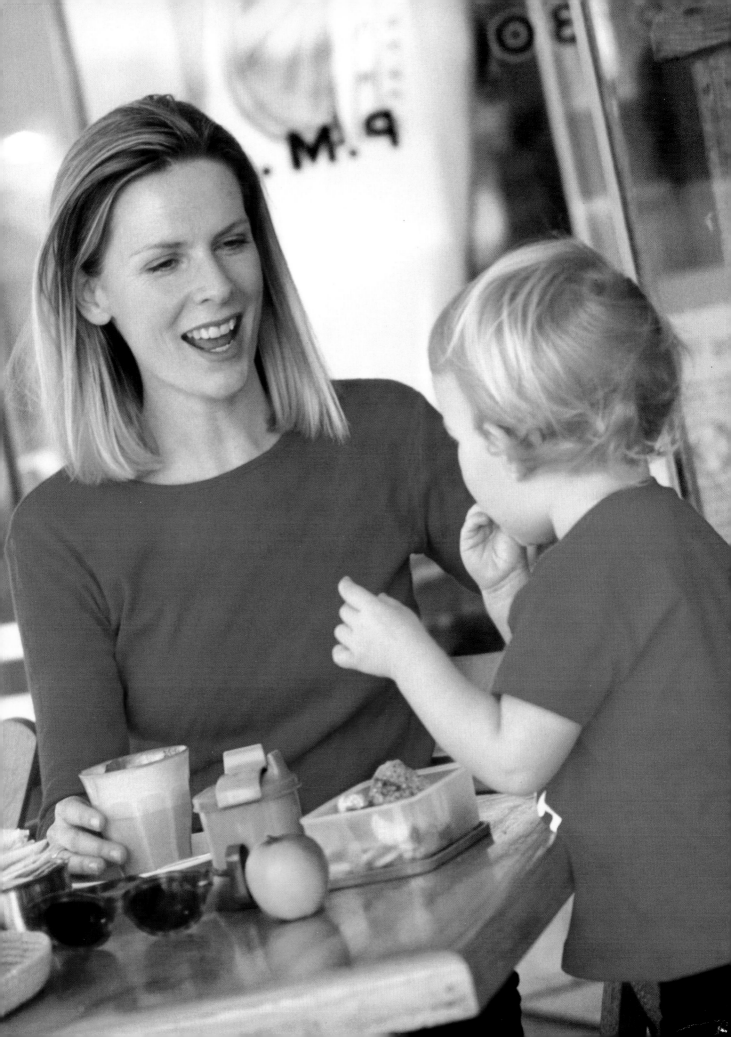

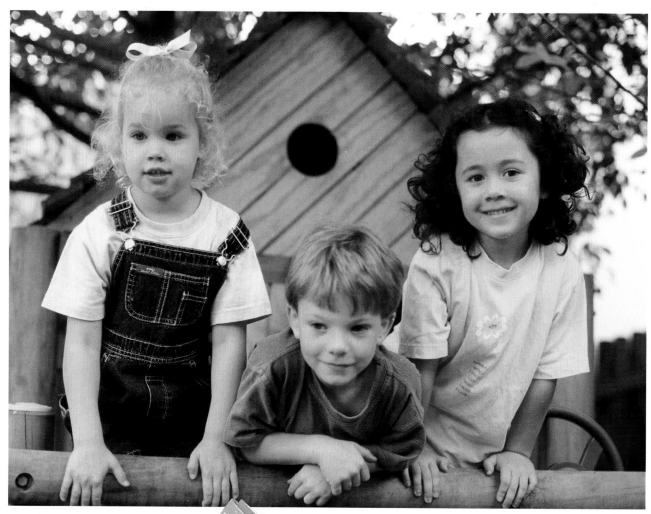

## The lunchbox

A plastic lunchbox is an ideal way of presenting food to a curious toddler, as well as being useful to transport a meal when the need arises.

Most preschools serve their own meals these days, so you will probably not need to pack lunch with the monotonous regularity that happens once school starts. But there are still sure to be lots of times when a packed lunchbox will come in handy, as well as providing fun and variety in your toddler's meals. Older preschoolers also love the idea of having their own "grown up" lunchbox, ready for school.

Some lunchboxes come with a fitted plastic drink bottle that doubles as a food container when filled with cold or frozen drink. This is ideal because it enables you to provide water or to dilute juice as you wish, but a cold juice box is a convenient, if more expensive, alternative.

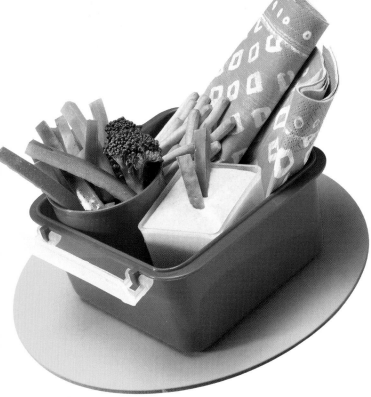

SMALL BREAD STICKS, VEGETABLE STICKS AND DIP

## Tempting children to lunch

• When packing a lunchbox, consider the age of the child as well as how long you need the food to keep before it is consumed – even the most valiant of eaters will probably suffer a loss of appetite when faced with The Soggy Tomato Sandwich.

• Preschoolers are far more likely to be tempted by lots of small packages of different things than one big sandwich and a piece of fruit. In fact, it is a rare toddler indeed who will eat a whole piece of fruit, so cut it into smaller portions, wrapping them individually to prevent browning – or try mini-containers of grapes or melon cubes.

• Dried fruit is an alternative to soggy or wasted fresh fruit and there is a wide variety available both from supermarkets and health food stores.

• Cut sandwiches into interesting shapes using a cookie cutter.

• As a change from your usual loaf, roll grated salad ingredients into cracker bread and cut into mini-rolls.

• Create a triple-decker effect, using brown and white bread alternately with simple fillings, such as ham, cream cheese and lettuce. Slice sandwich into fingers and pack on their sides so that the child can see the layers.

• Make sliced bread into "rolls" by removing crusts and flattening slightly. Spread with a simple filling, such as Vegemite or Marmite (see Glossary), peanut butter or ham, and roll up. Wrap tightly in plastic wrap, refrigerate, then slice into thin rounds when cold.

• Instead of serving a sandwich, cut favorite foods, such as bread, tomato, cheese, ham and celery, into bite-size bits and serve in a small lettuce-leaf cup as a finger-food salad.

• Mix chopped leftover cooked potatoes with mayonnaise. Spoon into a lettuce leaf with cold cooked chicken or chopped hard-boiled egg, tomato and other salad ingredients.

• Cold cooked rice tossed with a little French dressing and chopped celery, sweet red bell pepper, golden raisins, orange segments and chopped cooked chicken makes a delicious change.

• Make interesting salads from cold noodles or pasta – just add bite-size bits of the foods you know your toddler enjoys.

• Serve cubes of mild cheese with a small bowl of chopped fruit.

• Serve crackers or small bread sticks with dips for a change from bread.

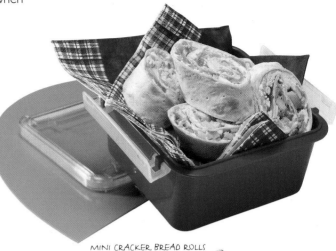

*popular toddler lunch boxes*

MINI CRACKER BREAD ROLLS

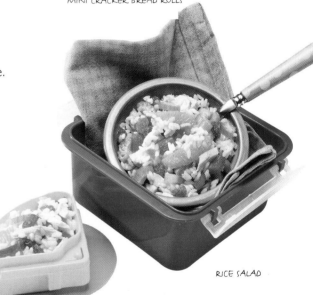

RICE SALAD

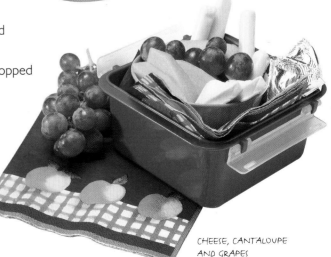

CHEESE, CANTALOUPE AND GRAPES

## Food to go

Wherever you are traveling, carrying prepared snacks will save you having to resort to expensive and nutritionally dubious fast food.

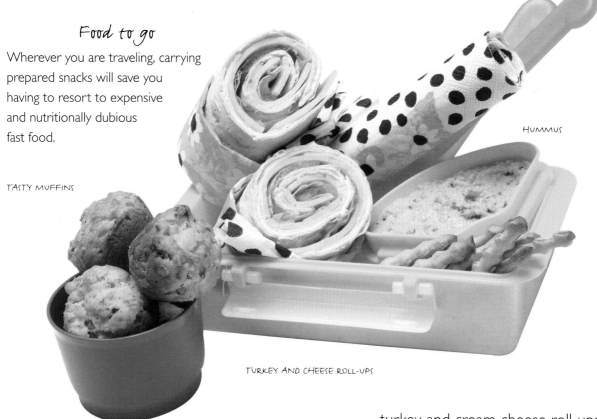

TASTY MUFFINS

HUMMUS

TURKEY AND CHEESE ROLL-UPS

### tasty muffins

**2 cups self-rising flour**
**1/2 cup finely chopped ham**
**1/2 cup coarsely grated cheddar cheese**
**1/4 cup finely chopped mushrooms**
**1 small sweet red bell pepper, chopped finely**
**1 1/2 tablespoons finely chopped fresh parsley**
**1/2 cup butter, melted**
**1 cup milk**
**1 egg, beaten lightly**

Grease three 12-cup mini (2-tablespoon-capacity) muffin tins.

Combine flour, ham, cheese, mushrooms, bell pepper and parsley in large bowl. Stir in butter, milk and egg; do not overmix. Divide mixture among muffin cups. Bake at 400°F 15 minutes; turn onto wire rack to cool.

MAKES 30

**Storage** Covered, in refrigerator, up to 2 days
**Freeze** Suitable

### turkey and cream cheese roll-ups

**1 piece cracker bread**
**1 1/2 tablespoon spreadable cream cheese**
**3 slices smoked turkey**
**3 cheese slices**
**3 iceberg lettuce leaves**
**1 small plum tomato, sliced thinly**

Spread bread with cream cheese. Place turkey, cheese, lettuce and tomato on cracker bread; roll tightly then cut into quarters.

MAKES 4 SERVINGS

*Best made on day of serving*

### hummus

**2 teaspoons lemon juice**
**1 clove garlic**
**1/2 teaspoon ground cumin**
**3/4 cup drained canned garbanzos**
**1/4 cup milk**
**1 teaspoon tahini**
**2 teaspoons finely chopped fresh cilantro**

Blend or process all ingredients until smooth. Serve with small bread sticks.

MAKES 1 1/2 CUPS

**Storage** Covered, in refrigerator, up to 2 days

## toddler ranch hand's lunch

*We used French onion dip in this recipe, but try other varieties
such as salmon or avocado.*

**1/2 small carrot**
**3 asparagus spears, trimmed**
**3 snow peas, trimmed**
**1 slice corned beef**
**1/2 cup (2 oz) cheddar cheese, cubed**
**1 small plum tomato, quartered**
**3 tablespoons packaged French onion dip**
**1 bread roll**

Cut carrot into sticks. Boil, steam or microwave carrot,
asparagus and snow peas, separately, until just tender; drain.
  Arrange all ingredients in lunchbox or on plate.

MAKES 1 SERVING

*Best made just before serving*

## muesli bar

*We suggest that only toddlers aged over three be given this as a treat.*

**1/2 cup butter**
**1/2 cup firmly packed brown sugar**
**1 1/2 tablespoons honey**
**2 cups rolled oats**
**1/4 cup sesame seeds, toasted**
**1/4 cup sunflower seeds, chopped finely**
**1/4 cup dried coconut, toasted**
**1/4 cup finely chopped pecans or walnuts**
**1/4 cup golden raisins**
**3 tablespoons unprocessed bran**
**1/2 teaspoon ground cinnamon**

Grease 9" x 12" cake pan. Combine butter, sugar
and honey in medium pan; stir over low heat until sugar
dissolves. Stir in remaining ingredients. Press mixture into
prepared pan; bake at 350°F about 25 minutes or until
browned lightly. While still warm, cut through bar into
15 pieces; cool in pan.

MAKES 15

**Storage**  Airtight container, up to 4 days

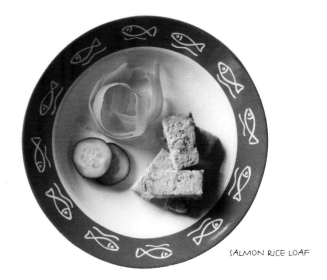

SALMON RICE LOAF

## salmon rice loaf

*You will need a little over 1/3 cup uncooked short grain rice for this recipe.*

**15-oz can red salmon, drained, flaked**
**1 cup cooked short grain rice**
**1 cup fresh breadcrumbs**
**1 cup sour cream**
**1 small onion, chopped finely**
**3 eggs, beaten lightly**
**1 1/2 tablespoons finely chopped fresh parsley**
**1 teaspoon Dijon mustard**
**1 teaspoon finely grated lemon rind**
**3 tablespoons lemon juice**

Grease 6" x 10" loaf pan, line bottom with parchment paper.
Combine all ingredients in large bowl; mix well. Spoon mixture
into prepared pan, smooth top; bake at 400°F about 1 hour or
until set. Let stand 10 minutes; turn onto wire rack.

MAKES 8 SERVINGS

**Storage**  Covered, in refrigerator, up to 2 days

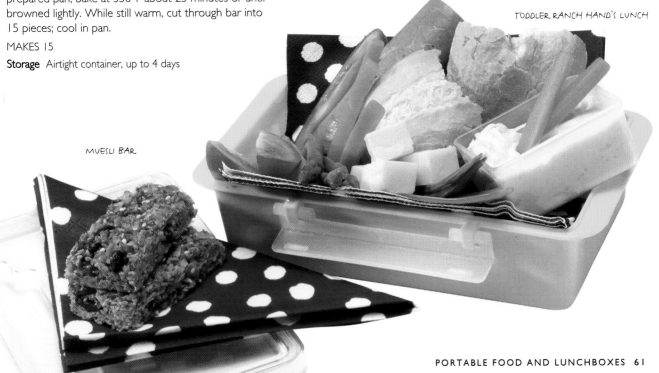

TODDLER RANCH HAND'S LUNCH

MUESLI BAR

## Pint-sized picnic fare

They might be meant for toddlers but adults will also enjoy these delicious and easily transported picnic foods – just make enough for the whole family.

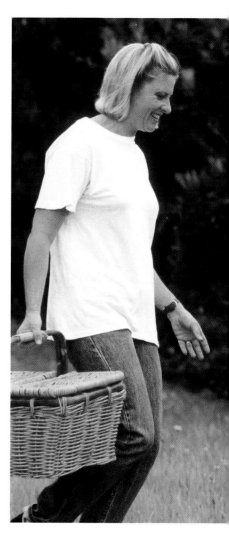

## Mediterranean meatballs

*If fresh herbs are not available, use 1/2 teaspoon each dried mint and basil.*

**I lb ground beef**
**I medium
   zucchini, grated
   coarsely**
**I medium
   carrot, grated
   coarsely**
**I small onion,
   chopped finely**
**1/2 cup fresh breadcrumbs**
**3 tablespoons catsup**
**I 1/2 tablespoons finely chopped
   fresh mint**
**I 1/2 tablespoons finely chopped
   fresh basil**
**I egg, beaten lightly**

YOGURT CUCUMBER SAUCE
**I cucumber,
   peeled, seeded**
**1/2 cup yogurt**

Combine all meatball ingredients in medium bowl; using hands, roll rounded tablespoons of mixture into balls. Place on greased baking sheet; bake, uncovered, at 350°F about 20 minutes or until cooked through. Serve with Yogurt Cucumber Sauce.

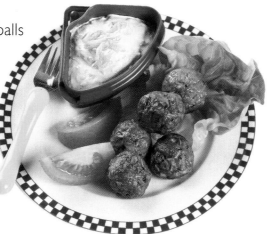

MEDITERRANEAN MEATBALLS

**Yogurt Cucumber Sauce** Grate cucumber coarsely; place in strainer, allow to drain 20 minutes then combine with yogurt in small bowl.

MAKES 35

**Storage** Covered, in refrigerator, up to 2 days
**Freeze** Uncooked meatballs suitable

## potato tortilla

*This is a Spanish dish which is usually cut into wedges and eaten cold – so it is great for a picnic.*

**3 tablespoons olive oil**
**2 medium potatoes,
   sliced thinly**
**I small onion,
   chopped finely**
**6 eggs, beaten lightly**

Heat I 1/2 tablespoons of the oil in 10-inch non-stick skillet; cook potatoes and onion, stirring, about 5 minutes or until potatoes are tender. Remove from skillet; combine in medium bowl with eggs.

Heat remaining oil in same skillet; pour in egg mixture. Cook, tilting skillet, over medium heat until eggs are almost set. Place skillet under heated broiler until top is browned lightly. Serve hot or cold, cut into wedges.

MAKES 4 TO 8 SERVINGS

**Storage** Covered, in refrigerator, up to 2 days

## golden raisin slice

**1/2 cup butter (4 oz)**
**1/2 cup superfine sugar**
**2 eggs**
**1/2 cup self-rising flour**
**1/2 cup all-purpose flour**
**I 1/2 cups golden raisins**

Grease 9" × 12" cake pan, line bottom with parchment paper. Beat butter and sugar in small bowl with electric mixer until light and fluffy. Add eggs, I at a time, beating well between additions. Stir in flours and raisins; spread mixture into prepared pan. Bake at 350°F about 25 minutes; cool in pan. Cut into fingers to serve.

**Storage** Airtight container, up to 4 days

## submarine sandwich

Split a small French bread loaf or long soft roll in half lengthwise; remove and discard some of the soft center. Fill hollowed-out bread with whatever sandwich filling your children like best; slice and wrap in plastic until ready to eat.

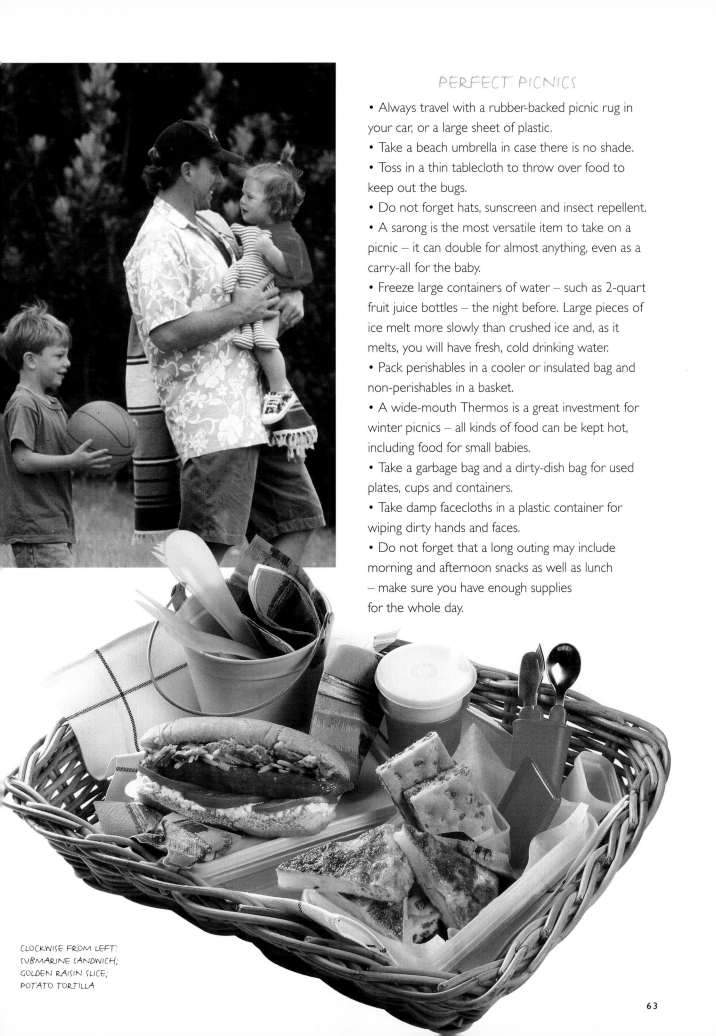

- Always travel with a rubber-backed picnic rug in your car, or a large sheet of plastic.
- Take a beach umbrella in case there is no shade.
- Toss in a thin tablecloth to throw over food to keep out the bugs.
- Do not forget hats, sunscreen and insect repellent.
- A sarong is the most versatile item to take on a picnic – it can double for almost anything, even as a carry-all for the baby.
- Freeze large containers of water – such as 2-quart fruit juice bottles – the night before. Large pieces of ice melt more slowly than crushed ice and, as it melts, you will have fresh, cold drinking water.
- Pack perishables in a cooler or insulated bag and non-perishables in a basket.
- A wide-mouth Thermos is a great investment for winter picnics – all kinds of food can be kept hot, including food for small babies.
- Take a garbage bag and a dirty-dish bag for used plates, cups and containers.
- Take damp facecloths in a plastic container for wiping dirty hands and faces.
- Do not forget that a long outing may include morning and afternoon snacks as well as lunch – make sure you have enough supplies for the whole day.

CLOCKWISE FROM LEFT:
SUBMARINE SANDWICH;
GOLDEN RAISIN SLICE;
POTATO TORTILLA

## crispy drumettes

**12 large (3 lb) chicken wings**
**¼ cup all-purpose flour**
**1 egg, beaten lightly**
**¼ cup milk**
**¾ cup finely crushed tortilla chips**
**1½ tablespoons olive oil**

Remove and discard tip from each wing; cut wings in half at joint. Using meaty half of wing (freeze remaining half), hold small end of each piece, trim around bone to cut meat free; cut, scrape and push meat towards large end. Pull skin and meat down over end of bone; each wing piece will resemble a baby drumstick.

Roll wings in flour, shake off excess; dip in combined egg and milk then in tortilla chips. Place wings on greased baking sheet; drizzle with oil. Bake, uncovered, at 350°F about 40 minutes or until wings are cooked and browned. Serve hot or cold.

MAKES 12

**Storage**  Covered, in refrigerator, up to 2 days

## cheese and spinach pie

*Two 10-ounce packages of frozen spinach, thawed and squeezed until excess moisture is eliminated, can be substituted for fresh spinach.*

**1½ tablespoons olive oil**
**1 small onion, chopped finely**
**3 green onions, chopped finely**
**1 clove garlic, crushed**
**1 lb spinach, trimmed, chopped**
**1 cup cottage cheese**
**½ cup feta cheese, crumbled**
**¼ cup finely grated parmesan cheese**
**¼ cup finely chopped fresh parsley**
**4 eggs, beaten lightly**
**½ teaspoon dry mustard**
**¼ teaspoon ground nutmeg**
**8 sheets filo pastry**
**¼ cup olive oil, extra**

Grease 8" x 12" rectangular cake pan. Heat oil in large pan; cook onion and garlic, stirring, until onion is soft. Add spinach; cook, stirring, until just wilted. Transfer to large bowl; stir in cheeses, parsley, eggs, mustard and nutmeg.

To prevent pastry from drying out, cover with damp cloth until ready to use. Brush 1 sheet of pastry with oil, fold in half horizontally, ease into prepared pan; repeat with 3 more pastry sheets. Pour spinach mixture over pastry in pan; repeat brushing with oil, folding and placing remaining 4 sheets of pastry over spinach mixture, tucking edges down into side of pan. Brush top with oil; using sharp knife, mark uncooked pie into 8 portions. Bake at 400°F about 30 minutes or until set.

SERVES 8

**Storage**  Covered, in refrigerator, up to 2 days

CLOCKWISE FROM TOP LEFT: CHEESE AND SPINACH PIE; SALMON RICE LOAF (PAGE 61); CARROT AND PINEAPPLE CAKE; EASY SUMMER SALAD; AND CRISPY DRUMETTES

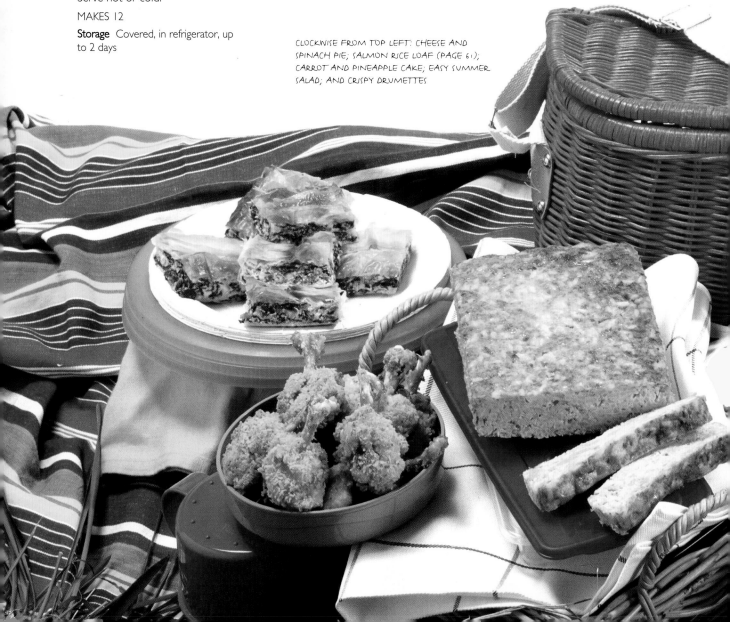

## easy summer salad

**6 small potatoes,
  chopped coarsely**
**2 medium apples, peeled,
  chopped coarsely**
**1/2 cup golden raisins**
**8 oz cherry tomatoes
  (about 16), halved**
**1/4 cup bottled coleslaw dressing**
**1/4 cup yogurt**

Boil, steam or microwave potato until tender; drain. Combine cooled potato in large bowl with remaining ingredients; toss gently.

SERVES 6 TO 8

*Best made just before serving*

## carrot and pineapple cake

*You will need 2 medium carrots
for this cake.*

**1 3/4 cups self-rising flour**
**1/2 teaspoon baking soda**
**1 teaspoon ground cinnamon**
**3/4 cup superfine sugar**
**1/2 cup ground almonds**
**2/3 cup dried coconut**
**3 eggs, beaten lightly**
**1/2 cup vegetable oil**
**3/4 cup yogurt**
**1 1/2 cups coarsely grated carrot**
**1/2 cup drained canned crushed
  pineapple**

Grease deep 8-inch square cake pan, line bottom with parchment paper. Combine flour, soda and cinnamon in large bowl with sugar, almonds and coconut. Stir in remaining ingredients. Spread mixture into prepared pan; bake at 350°F 1 hour. Let cake stand for 10 minutes; turn onto wire rack to cool. Just before serving, dust with powdered sugar.

**Storage**  Airtight container, in refrigerator, up to 4 days
**Freeze**  Suitable

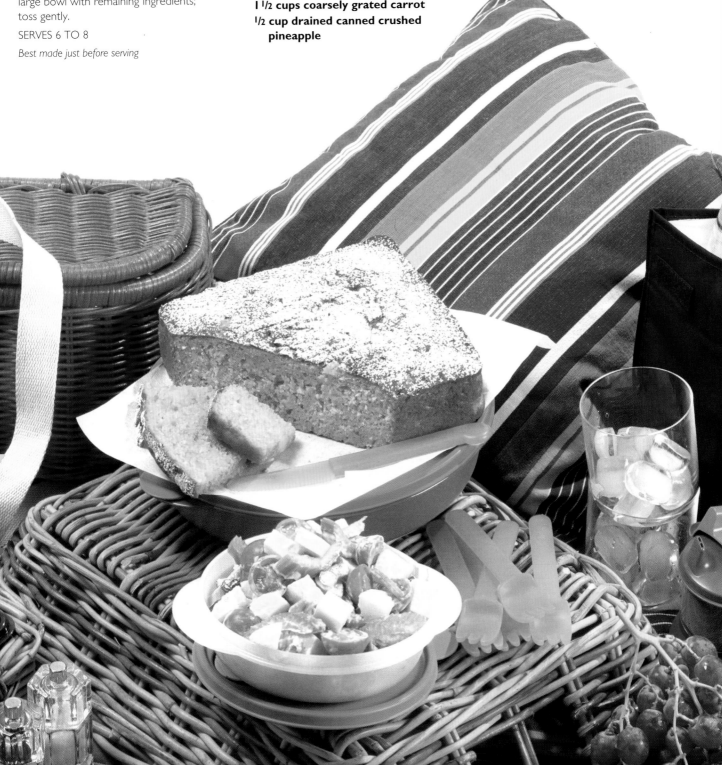

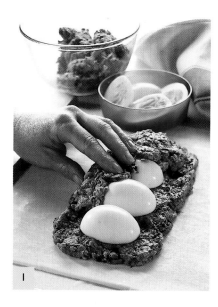

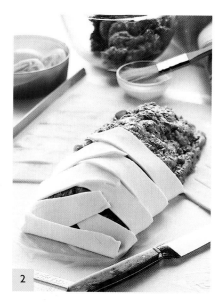

## sausage twist

**1 lb ground sausage**
**1 cup fresh breadcrumbs**
**2 green onions, chopped finely**
**3 tablespoons catsup**
**2 teaspoons Worcestershire**
  **sauce**
**1 1/2 tablespoons fruit chutney**
**3 tablespoons finely chopped**
  **fresh parsley**
**1 clove garlic, crushed**
**1/2 teaspoon sweet paprika**
**1/2 teaspoon apple-pie spice**
**2 sheets prepackaged**
  **piecrust pastry**
**4 hard-boiled eggs, halved**
**1 1/2 tablespoons milk**

Combine ground sausage, breadcrumbs, onion, catsup, Worcestershire sauce, chutney, parsley, garlic and spices in large bowl. Place each sheet of pastry on a separate greased and parchment-lined baking sheet. Spread a quarter of sausage mixture along the center of each pastry sheet; place 4 egg halves on top of each.

### STEP 1
Using wet hand, gently press remaining ground sausage mixture over egg halves.

### STEP 2
Make diagonal cuts on pastry on each side of the filling at 3/4-inch intervals. Lift alternate strips of pastry over filling to resemble braid; tuck ends under, brush pastry braids all over with milk. Bake at 400°F about 35 minutes or until browned lightly; lift onto wire rack to cool.

MAKES 4 TO 6 SERVINGS

**Storage** Covered, in refrigerator, up to 2 days

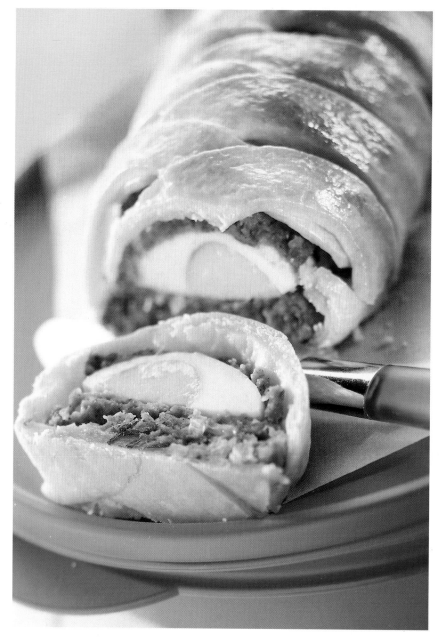

*SAUSAGE TWIST*

## mini suppli

*Suppli is the Italian name of these delicious deep-fried balls of rice with their core of melted mozzarella.*

**2 teaspoons butter**
**1 small onion, grated**
**1 clove garlic, crushed**
**1/3 cup short grain rice**
**2/3 cup chicken stock**
**1 1/2 tablespoons tomato paste**
**3 tablespoons finely grated parmesan cheese**
**1 egg, beaten lightly**
**1 1/2 oz mozzarella cheese (1/3 cup)**
**1/4 cup packaged breadcrumbs**
**vegetable oil, for deep-frying**

Melt butter in small pan; cook onion and garlic, stirring, until onion is soft. Add rice; stir until coated with butter. Add stock and tomato paste, bring to boil; simmer over low heat, covered, about 10 minutes or until rice is tender. Quickly stir parmesan and egg into rice; cool.

Cut mozzarella cheese in 12 even-size cubes. Using your hand, mold 1 1/2 tablespoons of rice mixture around each mozzarella cube to make ball shape. Gently toss rice balls in breadcrumbs, cover; refrigerate about 2 hours or until firm.

Heat oil in large deep pan; deep-fry suppli, in batches, until browned lightly, drain on paper towels.

MAKES 12

*Best made just before serving*

MINI SUPPLI

## salmon quichettes

**1 sheet prepackaged piecrust pastry**
**1/2 cup grated cheddar cheese**
**4 oz can red salmon, drained, flaked**
**1/2 cup milk**
**1 egg**

Cut pastry into nine 3-inch rounds; press pastry rounds into cups of greased muffin tin or tart pan. Divide combined cheese and salmon among pastry shells.

Whisk together milk and egg in small bowl; pour enough into each pastry shell to cover filling. Bake at 350°F about 20 minutes or until filling is set. Cool 5 minutes before removing from pan.

MAKES 9

*Best made just before serving*

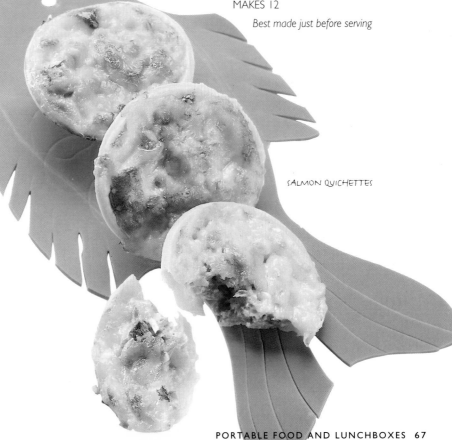

SALMON QUICHETTES

## scaloppine fingers

**2 thin veal steaks (about 6 oz)**
**3 tablespoons all-purpose flour**
**1 egg, beaten lightly**
**3/4 cup packaged breadcrumbs**
**vegetable oil, for frying**

Coat veal in flour, shake off excess; dip into egg, then coat in breadcrumbs. Place in single layer on tray, cover; refrigerate 30 minutes. Fry veal in hot oil until browned both sides and cooked through. Serve sliced into fingers.

MAKES 4 SERVINGS

*Best made just before serving*

BBQ CHOPSS

FROM BACK: BEANY LETTUCE
ROLL-UPS AND SCALOPPINE FINGERS

☺ TIP Toddlers love to dip, so try serving these crunchy veal fingers with yogurt, or catsup, barbecue or sweet and sour sauce.

## beany lettuce roll-ups

*You will need 2/3 cup of uncooked short grain rice for this recipe.*

**2 cups cooked short grain rice**
**1 cup canned mixed beans, drained, rinsed**
**1 small apple, peeled, chopped finely**
**1 celery stalk, chopped finely**
**1 green onion, chopped finely**
**1/4 cup golden raisins**
**1/4 cup French dressing**
**6 large romaine lettuce leaves**

Combine rice, beans, apple, celery, onion, raisins and dressing in a large bowl. Divide filling mixture among lettuce leaves; roll securely to form parcels.

MAKES 6

*Best rolled just before serving*

**Storage** Filling, covered, in refrigerator up to 2 days

## cracker "nachos"

**6 oz small crackers**
**7 oz prepared avocado dip**
**1/2 cup canned kidney beans, drained**
**1 small tomato, chopped finely**
**1/2 cup coarsely grated cheddar cheese**

Arrange crackers on serving plate. Spoon dip and combined beans and tomato over the top; sprinkle with cheese, serve immediately.

MAKES 6 SERVINGS

☺ TIP You can use any small crackers, zwieback, mini-Ritz or tortilla chips if your toddler is old enough to chew properly.

## bbq chops

**6 lamb rib chops**
**1/4 cup barbecue sauce**
**1/4 cup plum sauce**

Trim lamb chops of excess fat; brush each chop with combined sauces. Cook chops on heated oiled griddle (or broiler or barbecue) until browned both sides and tender, brushing occasionally with remaining combined sauces. Pack cooled chops in lunch-box with salad and bread.

MAKES 6

*Best made just before serving*

**Storage** Covered, in refrigerator, up to 2 days

CRACKER "NACH(

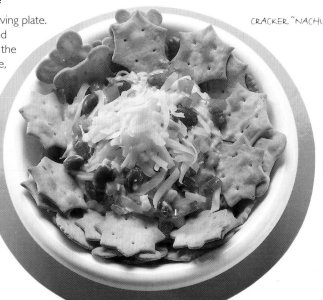

## vegetable and cheese tarts

**1 sheet prepackaged piecrust shortcrust pastry**
**1/2 small tomato, chopped finely**
**1/2 small carrot, chopped finely**
**1/2 small zucchini, chopped finely**
**1/4 cup drained canned kidney beans**
**3 tablespoons frozen peas, thawed**
**2/3 cup finely grated cheddar cheese**

Cut pastry into 3-inch rounds; press pastry rounds into greased cups of muffin tin or tart pan, prick well with skewer or fork. Bake at 400°F about 15 minutes or until browned lightly.

Meanwhile, combine tomato, carrot, zucchini, beans and peas in small bowl; divide mixture among tart shells, sprinkle cheese over top of each. Bake tarts at 350°F about 10 minutes or until the cheese melts.

MAKES 9

**Storage** Covered in refrigerator, up to 1 day

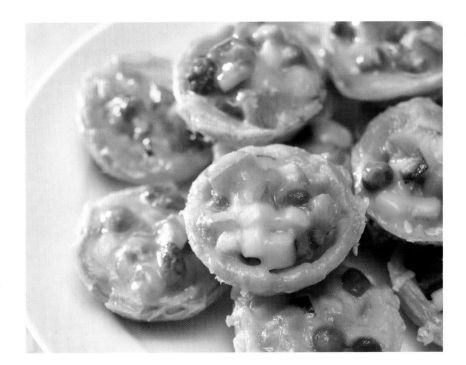

## chicken burritos

**1 1/4 cups coarsely chopped cooked chicken (about 1/2 lb)**
**1/4 cup mayonnaise**
**1/4 cup sour cream**
**3 flour tortillas (8-inches)**
**1 cup finely shredded lettuce**
**2 small tomatoes, chopped finely**
**1/2 cup coarsely grated cheddar cheese**

Combine chicken, mayonnaise and sour cream in medium bowl. Divide mixture, lettuce, tomato and cheese among tortillas; roll securely to enclose filling. Cut in half to serve.

MAKES 6

*Best made just before serving*

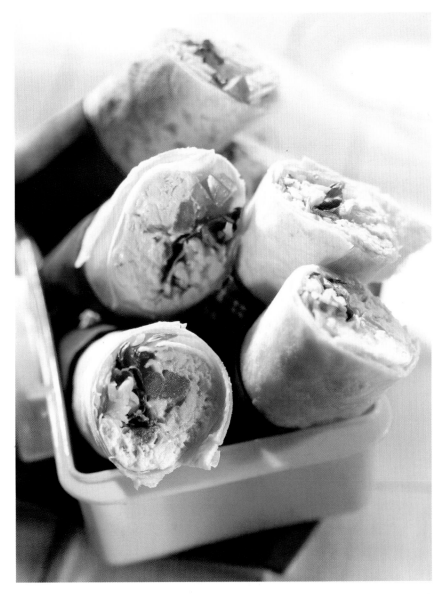

RIGHT FROM TOP: VEGETABLE AND CHEESE TARTS; CHICKEN BURRITOS

## Fruit, the all-time favorite

Chopped and fresh or incorporated into muffins and cakes, fruit is versatile, nutritious and always popular.

### little pear and cinnamon cakes

**I medium pear**
**1/2 cup vegetable oil**
**1/3 cup superfine sugar**
**I egg**
**1/2 cup all-purpose flour**
**1/2 cup self-rising flour**
**1/4 teaspoon ground cinnamon**
**1/2 teaspoon superfine sugar, extra**

Grease two 12-cup (2-tablespoon capacity) mini muffin tins. Peel and halve pear, remove and discard core; chop into 3/8-inch pieces. Whisk oil, sugar and egg together in medium bowl.

Add flours and pear; stir until just combined. Drop rounded tablespoons of mixture into each pan cup; sprinkle with combined cinnamon and extra superfine sugar. Bake at 400°F about 15 minutes. Turn onto wire rack; serve warm or cold.

MAKES 24

**Storage** Airtight container, up to 3 days

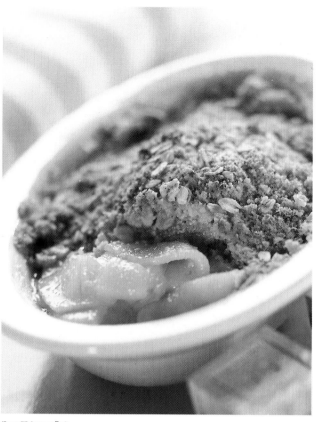

FRUIT CRUMBLE

### fruit crumble

**I small pear**
**I small apple**
**2 teaspoons superfine sugar**
**1/2 cup wholewheat flour**
**1/4 cup butter, chopped coarsely**
**1/4 cup firmly packed**
**brown sugar**
**I 1/2 tablespoons rolled oats**
**dash apple-pie spice**

Peel, core and thinly slice pear and apple; place in greased shallow 2-cup capacity ovenproof dish, sprinkle superfine sugar over the top. Place flour in small bowl, rub in butter until mixture resembles breadcrumbs; stir in brown sugar and oats. Sprinkle over fruit, dust with spice. Bake 350°F about 25 minutes or until just browned.

MAKES
2 SERVINGS

**Storage** Covered, in refrigerator, up to 2 days

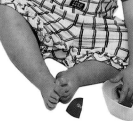

LITTLE PEAR AND CINNAMON CAKES

# fruit fantastic

Do not just chop it and serve it – with a little extra thought, fruit will tempt even the fussiest eater – and with so much to choose from, something is sure to appeal.

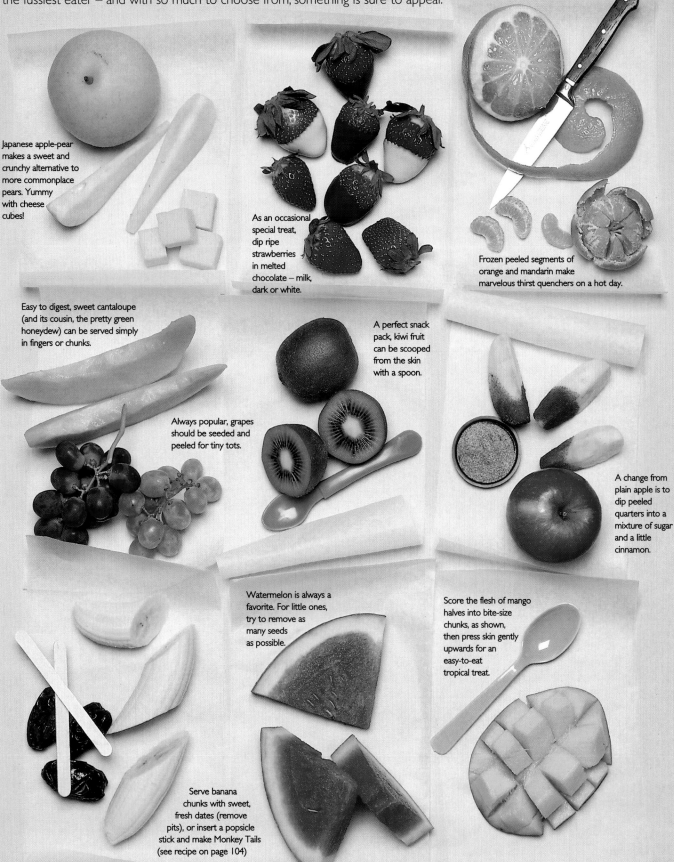

Japanese apple-pear makes a sweet and crunchy alternative to more commonplace pears. Yummy with cheese cubes!

As an occasional special treat, dip ripe strawberries in melted chocolate – milk, dark or white.

Frozen peeled segments of orange and mandarin make marvelous thirst quenchers on a hot day.

Easy to digest, sweet cantaloupe (and its cousin, the pretty green honeydew) can be served simply in fingers or chunks.

A perfect snack pack, kiwi fruit can be scooped from the skin with a spoon.

Always popular, grapes should be seeded and peeled for tiny tots.

A change from plain apple is to dip peeled quarters into a mixture of sugar and a little cinnamon.

Watermelon is always a favorite. For little ones, try to remove as many seeds as possible.

Score the flesh of mango halves into bite-size chunks, as shown, then press skin gently upwards for an easy-to-eat tropical treat.

Serve banana chunks with sweet, fresh dates (remove pits), or insert a popsicle stick and make Monkey Tails (see recipe on page 104)

## rock cakes

**2 cups self-rising flour**
**1/4 teaspoon ground cinnamon**
**1/3 cup butter, chopped coarsely**
**1/3 cup superfine sugar**
**I cup golden raisins**
**1/2 cup milk, approximately**
**I egg, beaten lightly**
**I 1/2 tablespoons superfine**
**sugar, extra**

Sift flour and cinnamon into large bowl; rub in butter, stir in sugar and golden raisins. Stir in egg, then enough milk to mix to a moist but firm dough; drop heaped tablespoons of mixture 2 inches apart onto greased baking sheets. Sprinkle a little extra superfine sugar over top of each cake; bake at 400°F about 15 minutes or until browned lightly. Loosen cakes; cool on trays.

MAKES 18

**Storage** Airtight container, up to 3 days

## apricot bars

*If there are any large pieces of nuts in the muesli, chop finely to avoid the risk of choking.*

**3/4 cup butter**
**3 tablespoons golden syrup**
**or honey**
**1/4 cup self-rising flour**
**1/4 cup all-purpose flour**
**1/2 cup natural muesli**
**1/2 cup brown sugar**
**1/2 cup finely chopped**
**dried apricots**
**1/4 cup golden raisins**
**1/4 cup rolled oats**
**1/4 cup dried coconut**
**2 eggs, beaten lightly**

Grease 9" x 12" cake pan; line bottom with parchment paper.

Combine butter and syrup in small pan; stir over low heat until butter melts. Combine sifted flours, muesli, sugar, apricots, raisins, oats and coconut together in large bowl; stir in eggs and cooled butter mixture.

Press mixture into prepared pan; bake at 350°F 25 minutes. Cool in pan; cut into fingers before serving.

**Storage** Airtight container, up to 4 days

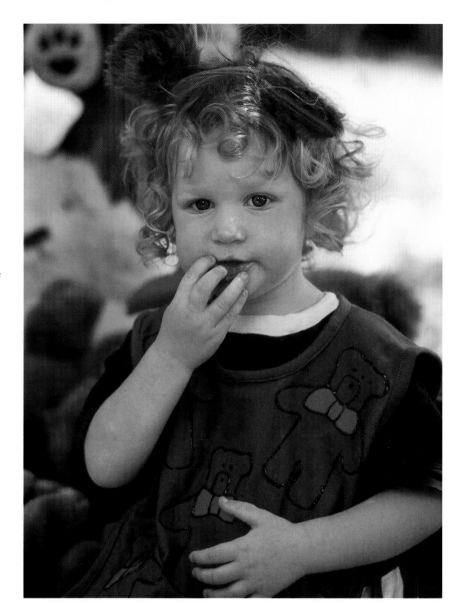

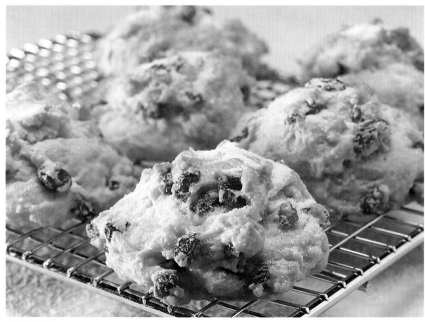

ROCK CAKES

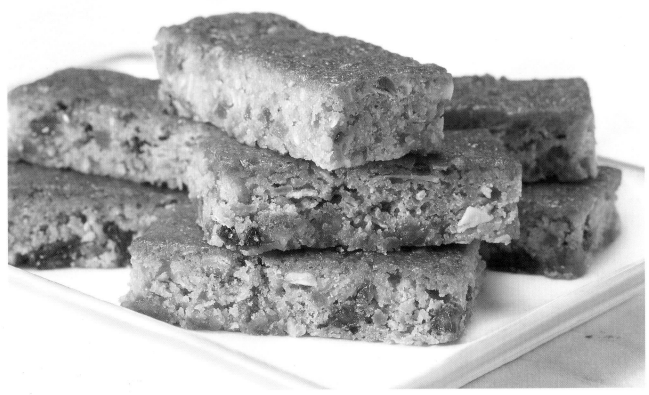

*APRICOT BARS*

## chunky chocolate cookies

**1 egg**
**¹/₂ cup firmly packed brown sugar**
**¹/₄ cup vegetable oil**
**²/₃ cup all-purpose flour**
**¹/₂ cup self-rising flour**
**¹/₄ teaspoon baking soda**
**3¹/₂ oz dark chocolate, melted**
**³/₄ cup dark chocolate patties**

CHOCOLATE ICING
**1¹/₂ tablespoons, melted**
**3 oz dark chocolate, melted**
**²/₃ cup powdered sugar**
**2 teaspoons milk, approximately**

Beat egg and sugar in medium bowl with electric mixer about 1 minute or until mixture changes color. Stir in oil and sifted dry ingredients then cooled melted chocolate (mixture will be soft). Cover, refrigerate 1 hour.

Roll heaped teaspoons of mixture into balls; place 2 inches apart on greased baking sheets. Bake at 400°F about 8 minutes or until cracked and slightly firm. Let stand on trays 5 minutes before turning onto wire racks to cool.

Spread top of each cookie with Chocolate Icing and top with dark chocolate patties. Dust with powdered sugar, if desired.

**Chocolate Icing** Combine cooled butter and chocolate with sifted powdered sugar in small bowl. Stir in enough milk to make a soft paste.

MAKES ABOUT 3 DOZEN

**Storage** Airtight container, up to 4 days

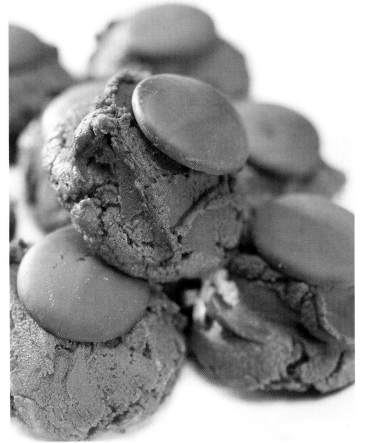

*CHUNKY CHOCOLATE COOKIES*

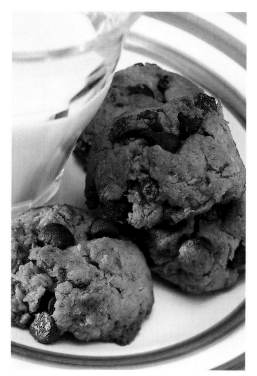

CRUNCHY COOKIES

## crunchy cookies

**¹/₃ cup butter**
**¹/₄ cup honey**
**3 tablespoons golden syrup
  or honey**
**1 cup self-rising flour**
**1 cup dried coconut**
**1 cup corn flakes**
**¹/₂ cup golden raisins**
**¹/₂ cup dark chocolate chips**

Combine butter, honey and golden syrup in medium pan; stir over heat until butter melts. Cool 5 minutes; stir in remaining ingredients, mix well. Drop rounded tablespoons of mixture about 2 inches apart onto baking sheets; bake at 350°F about 12 minutes. Let stand 5 minutes; turn onto wire racks to cool.

MAKES ABOUT 2 DOZEN

**Storage** Airtight container, up to 1 week

## lemonade

**¹/₂ cup sugar**
**¹/₂ cup water**
**¹/₂ cup lemon juice**
**3 cups water, extra**

Combine sugar and water in small pan; stir over low heat, without boiling, until sugar dissolves. Bring to boil; simmer, uncovered, 2 minutes. Stir in lemon juice, let stand 30 minutes. Strain mixture into large pitcher, add extra water; refrigerate until required.

MAKES 4 CUPS

## fruit fizz

**8 oz trimmed watermelon,
  chopped coarsely**
**8 oz trimmed pineapple,
  chopped coarsely**
**2 small oranges, peeled,
  chopped coarsely**
**1 cup sparkling
  mineral water**

Blend or process watermelon, pineapple and orange until smooth; strain juice into large pitcher. Just before serving, stir in mineral water.

MAKES 3 CUPS

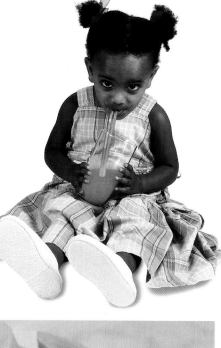

## quick-mix banana cake

*You need approximately 2 overripe bananas
for this recipe.*

**¹/₂ cup butter**
**³/₄ cup firmly packed
  brown sugar**
**2 eggs**
**¹/₃ cup sour cream**
**1 ¹/₂ cups self-rising flour**
**¹/₂ teaspoon baking soda**
**1 cup mashed banana**

LEMON ICING
**1 cup powdered sugar**
**1 tablespoon soft butter**
**1 ¹/₂ tablespoons lemon juice**
**2 teaspoons hot water,
  approximately**

Grease deep 8-inch square cake pan, line bottom with parchment paper.

Beat butter and sugar in small bowl with electric mixer until light and fluffy. Add eggs, sour cream, flour and soda; beat on low speed 1 minute. Stir in banana; spread mixture into prepared pan. Bake at 350°F 45 minutes. Let cake stand 10 minutes; turn onto wire rack. When cooled, top cake with Lemon Icing.

**Lemon Icing** Mix powdered sugar, butter and juice in small bowl; stir in enough water to make a spreadable consistency.

**Storage** Airtight container, in refrigerator, up to 4 days

QUICK-MIX BANANA CAKE

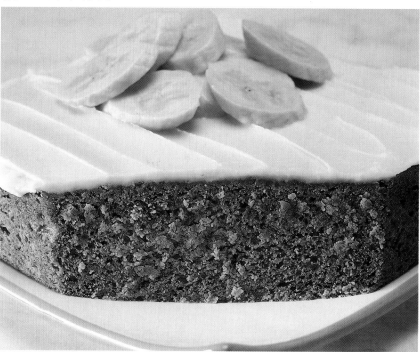

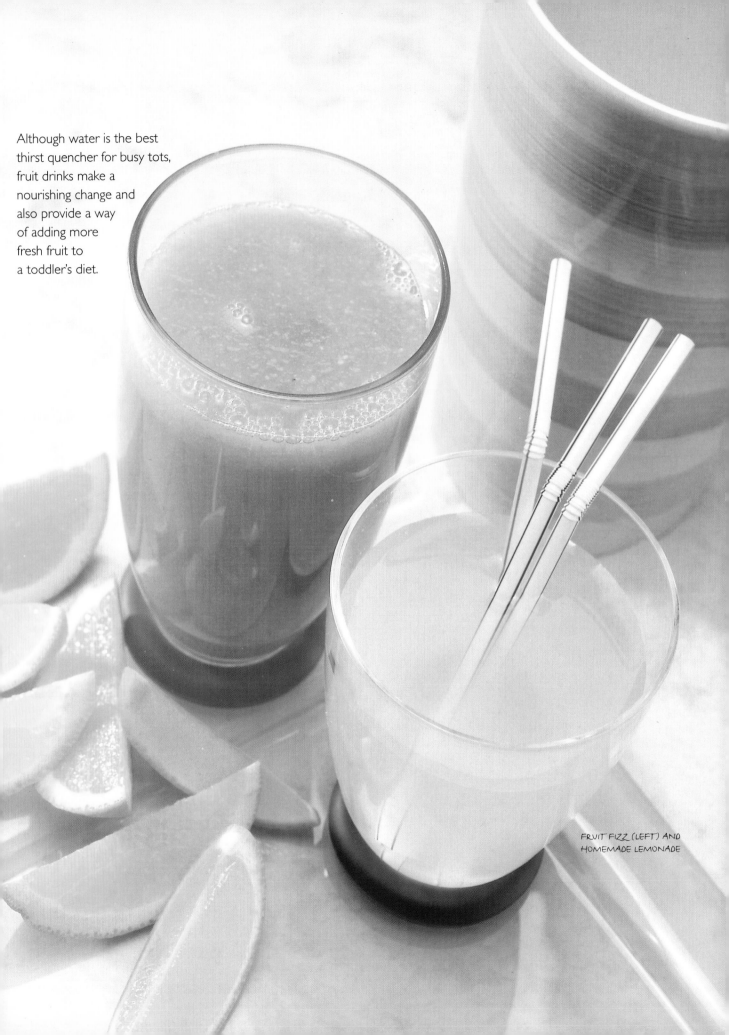

Although water is the best thirst quencher for busy tots, fruit drinks make a nourishing change and also provide a way of adding more fresh fruit to a toddler's diet.

FRUIT FIZZ (LEFT) AND HOMEMADE LEMONADE

# adapting family meals

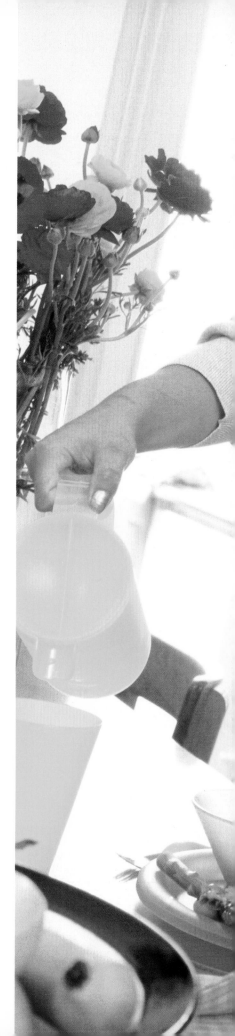

Delicate little purees are great when you are starting out, but there is no doubt that life becomes much easier when your toddler starts eating the same meals as you – unless, of course, your family lives on greasy take-out, in which case you might consider getting the rest of the family to eat what the toddler eats instead!

Adapting your family meals to suit the smallest member should really require very little extra effort. Obviously, you will need to cut things into bite-size pieces where appropriate, and for smaller toddlers you might still need to mash or grind some foods. But by and large, there is not much that a healthy toddler cannot eat, and most adaptation will be concerned with the texture or consistency rather than the ingredients. If your family meals involve curry, for instance, there is no reason why your toddler cannot have curry too – simply reserve his portion before you add the chili, then cut it up or puree as appropriate. This applies to all very strong tasting or salty foods – separate the child's portion before adding the "adult" ingredients, or add reduced amounts of strong spice to his so he gets used to the taste gradually. Do not assume that everything he eats needs to be completely bland, however – it does not, and if you fall into this trap you might find yourself with a very unadventurous eater on your hands.

Of course, you might already have one of these on your hands and at low moments you will have started to think you will be serving mashed banana sandwiches at his wedding – if he's lucky enough to find a partner who shares his hatred of anything green! Do not despair. Keep serving the foods that you know he likes, but offer a little taste of what you are having as well – this is easier if he is actually at the table with you. Do not insist that it is eaten, and do not make an issue when it is not. Eventually, he will realize that it is not a power game and that some of the things he has tried from your plate are actually quite nice!

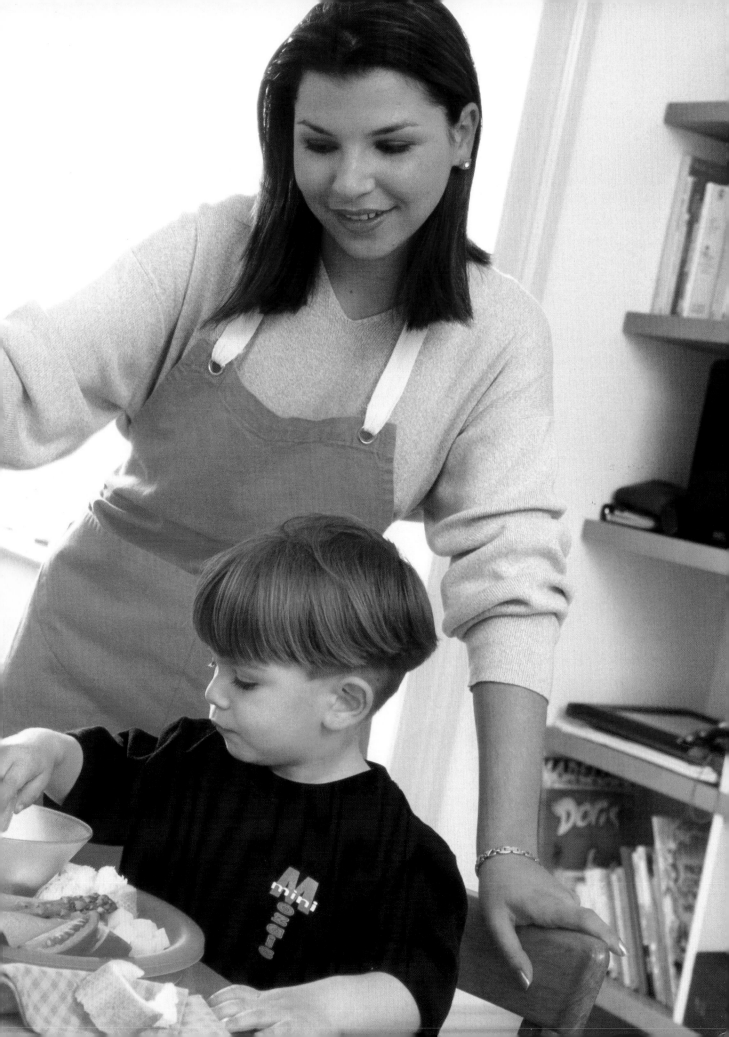

## Adjusting your favorite recipes

Remember to stick with a common sense approach and you will find it easy to adapt family meals to healthy toddler food. You might even find your own diet becomes a little healthier as well!

• For a perfectly balanced diet that includes everything a growing body needs, try to include some of each of the 5 food groups in each meal (see page 81), but be realistic as well and keep your eye on the big picture – if your toddler eats a variety of food over the course of a week or so, one or two fast-food meals are not going to result in malnutrition.

• When pureeing family food for younger babies, add a little boiled water, milk or salt-free stock to achieve the desired consistency.

• Consider the texture of what you are serving – tender meat is usually more attractive to a toddler, so bear this in mind when shopping.

• Reduce amounts of saturated fats, such as butter and cream, trim excess fat from meat and remove chicken skin. Remember, however, that some fat is an essential part of the diet of babies and toddlers – dairy products should be full-fat unless your doctor advises otherwise.

• Use herbs, garlic and onion to add flavor to your cooking instead of relying on salt.

• Steaming or microwaving vegetables retains more nutrients. If boiling, use only small amounts of water and reserve the cooking liquid for stock. If peeling your veggies, do so very thinly as most nutrients are located just below the skin.

• Use non-stick pans to avoid the need for too much oil.

• Bake meat on a rack so that excess fat drips away.

• Even if your toddler is not actually eating at the table with you, remember to save a little of your meal and refrigerate or freeze for serving to her at a later time.

Opposite we give a sample weekly menu planner to show you how easy it is to choose meals that all the family will enjoy. Mix and match as you choose – but remember, you are not running a restaurant!

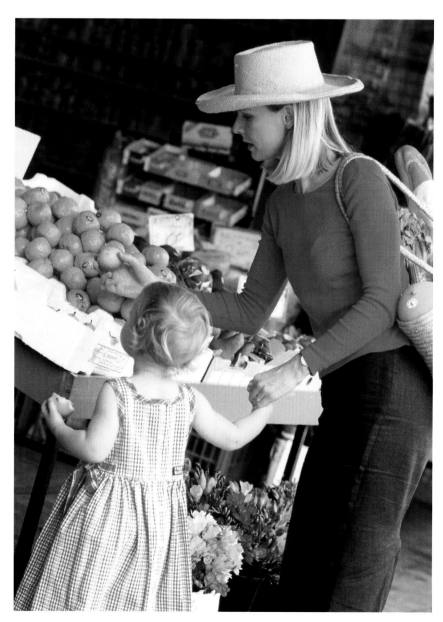

# sample weekly menu planner

## menu 1

MAIN  rice and vegetable soup
chive and bacon
quick bread

DESSERT  pear and ricotta strudel

## menu 2

MAIN  baked potato, ham
and cheese omelette
mixed green salad

DESSERT  rhubarb and berry compote

## menu 3

ENTREE  pumpkin and orange sweet
potato soup

MAIN  rack of lamb with
orange couscous
mixed green salad

## menu 4

ENTREE  rice paper veggie rolls

MAIN  glazed Thai chicken
steamed jasmine rice
mixed green salad

## menu 5

MAIN  fava bean and leek pasta
mixed green salad

DESSERT  baked orange cheesecake

## menu 6

MAIN  Atlantic salmon with
citrus butter sauce

DESSERT  quick-mix ice cream
and fruit salad

## menu 7

MAIN  sunday roast

DESSERT  citrus delicious

## Catering for vegetarians

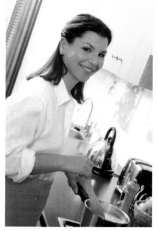

Choosing vegetarianism for your baby can involve problems unless you go into it armed with adequate knowledge. To ensure your baby gets a well-balanced diet, the first thing you should do is seek advice from your doctor or other health professional.

A well-nourished vegetarian mother can provide all the nutrients her baby requires for the first 6 months of life through breast milk (or infant formula). Milk is vital in the first year of a child's life, so if you are choosing vegetarianism, it is a good idea to breastfeed as long as possible. Fortified formula can be used and soy-based infant formulas are also available. It is after weaning when a child begins to eat family food that a strict vegetarian diet may cause problems.

If your vegetarian diet includes dairy products and eggs, it is fairly easy to provide all the nutritional requirements of a growing child. If fish can be added, providing adequate nourishment is even easier.

However, if you are a vegan (a diet of plant-based foods only), you may need to be a little more flexible when it comes to your baby's diet. This is because the strict regime of the vegan is really too bulky for a young child and may not include enough fat and protein for their many needs, particularly rapid growth.

When you are converting recipes to suit a vegetarian diet, do not simply remove the meat. Learn to combine two plant proteins (and increase the carbohydrate) so that the total mix of amino acids is sufficient to meet the child's needs. Meat substitutes can include legumes (such as baked beans), nutmeats, tofu or perhaps fish. Cheese or eggs can be added to many dishes for added protein and ground nuts – another source of protein – can be used to thicken sauces. Wherever possible, choose whole wheat pasta and breads and cook potatoes in their skin. Use milk, cheese, cottage cheese, yogurt and buttermilk as often as possible.

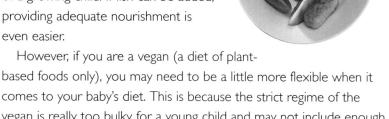

As with babies on a regular diet, introduce each new food one at a time and watch for an adverse reaction before starting the next new taste.

# Principles of a balanced diet

Today's food is rather different to that eaten 30 or even 20 years ago – it is more varied and interesting and, quite often, lighter. However, the fundamental principles of good nutrition remain the same.

Planning balanced meals for your toddler is as easy as remembering to include a little of each of the Five Food Groups in daily meals to ensure that you are supplying all the essential nutrients needed for growth and good health.

Many toddlers are extremely fussy about what they will and will not eat; others have periods where they eat almost nothing at all and are unlikely to be impressed by your great knowledge of nutrition. Try to remain flexible and keep things in perspective – if you look at your toddler's diet over a week, rather than becoming obsessed with its shortcomings over a day, you will probably find that malnutrition is not as imminent as you thought!

And remember, too, that many different combinations of foods can supply all the necessary nutrients, so that your child's diet might vary considerably from a playmate's yet still be perfectly healthy.

Do not forget the importance of water in any diet, and try to encourage your child to drink water from an early age. Fruit juice is a useful source of vitamin C, but a toddler does not need fruit juice every time she needs a drink – water is a far better thirst-quencher and will not cause tooth decay.

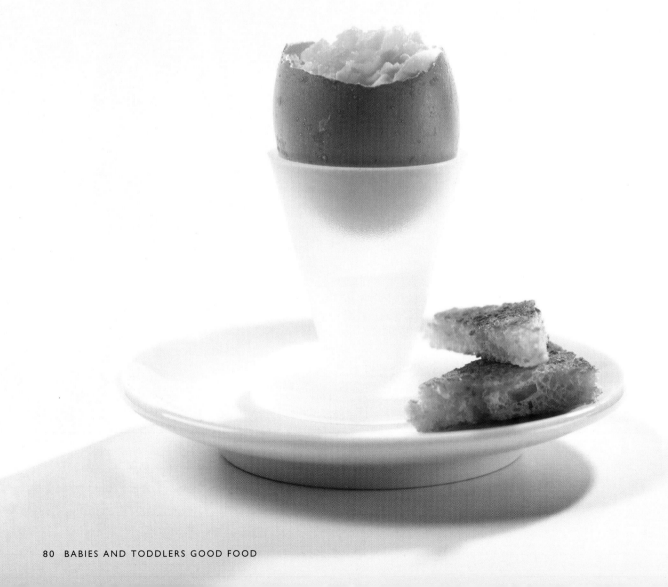

# The five food groups

### Breads, Grains and Cereals

This group provides carbohydrates for energy, as well as iron, B vitamins and fiber. Try for six or more servings per day; one serving is 1 slice of bread or 2 to 3 rye crackers or 1/2 cup cooked pasta or rice.

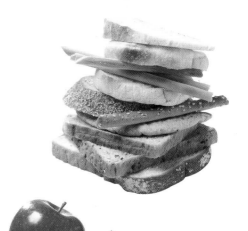

### Fruit, Vegetables and Salads

This group provides carbohydrates for energy, as well as iron and other minerals, calcium, several vitamins, including vitamin C, and fiber. Try for six or more servings per day; one serving is 1 piece of fruit or 1 medium potato or 1/2 cup vegetables or fruit salad or 1/2 cup juice.

### Milk and Dairy Products

This group provides calcium, protein, fat and several vitamins and minerals. Because babies require more fat than adults, the dairy products you serve to children should be full-fat unless medically advised. Three servings per day are recommended; one serving is 1 cup milk or 1 cup yogurt or 1 ounce (1/4 cup) cheese.

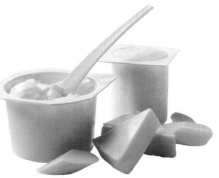

### Fish, Meat and Eggs

This group is the major supply of protein, essential for growth and the repair of body cells. It is very easy to supply adequate protein to children on non-restrictive diets but vegetarians need to take care that enough protein is provided from non-meat sources, such as eggs, dairy products, soy beans and legumes. One serving per day is recommended; one serving is 5 ounces fish or 4 ounces meat/chicken or 2 eggs.

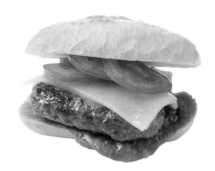

### Fats and Oils

Although this is the food group you should eat least of, it is still an important source of vitamins A and D and should never be excluded entirely. For health's sake, the best fats are unsaturated (such as vegetable oils and nuts) rather than saturated (such as butter, cream or animal fat). One serving per day is recommended; one serving is 1 teaspoon oil or 1 1/2 tablespoons nuts (do not give whole nuts to children under 5 years).

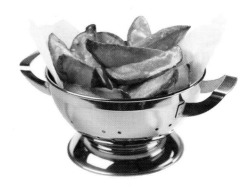

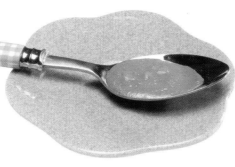

## rice and vegetable soup

- 1 1/2 tablespoons olive oil
- 1 medium yellow onion, chopped finely
- 1 trimmed celery stalk, chopped finely
- 1 medium carrot, chopped coarsely
- 4 cups vegetable stock
- 2 x 14 1/2 oz cans tomatoes
- 1 cup canned, mixed beans, rinsed, drained
- 1/2 cup long grain white rice
- 1/2 teaspoon sugar
- 3 tablespoons finely chopped fresh basil
- 1/3 cup finely grated parmesan cheese

RICE AND VEGETABLE SOUP, SHOWN PUREED FOR BABY

Heat oil in large pan; cook onion, celery and carrot, stirring, until onion is soft. Add stock, undrained crushed tomatoes, beans, rice and sugar. Bring to boil; simmer, uncovered, about 20 minutes or until rice is tender. Serve soup sprinkled with basil and cheese.

SERVES 4 TO 6

**Storage** Covered, in refrigerator, up to 2 days

**Freeze** Suitable

😊 FOR BABY Puree to the desired consistency

😊 FOR TODDLER Chop appropriately for stage of development

RICE AND VEGETABLE SOUP, TODDLER SERVING

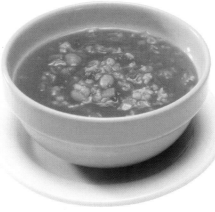

RICE AND VEGETABLE SOUP

## chive and bacon quick bread

- 2 slices bacon, chopped finely
- 2 cups self-rising flour
- 2 tablespoons butter
- 1/2 cup coarsely grated cheddar cheese
- 3 tablespoons finely chopped fresh chives
- 1/2 cup milk
- 1/2 cup water, aproximately

Cook bacon in medium heated oiled pan, stirring, until browned and crisp; drain on paper towels.

Place flour in large bowl, rub in butter, stir in cheese, chives and bacon. Add milk and enough water to mix to a soft, sticky dough. Turn dough onto floured surface, knead until smooth. Shape dough into 6-inch round; place on greased baking sheet. Mark 1/2-inch deep cross on top of dough; brush with a little extra milk, sprinkle with extra flour. Bake at 400°F 25 minutes.

*Best made on day of serving*

**Freeze** Suitable

😊 FOR BABY Serve a small portion of quick bread broken into tiny pieces

😊 FOR TODDLER Serve as above

CHIVE AND BACON QUICK BREAD

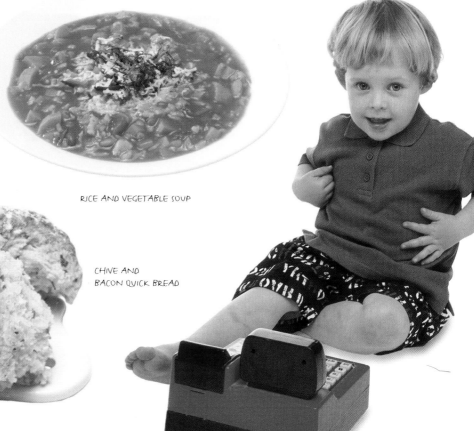

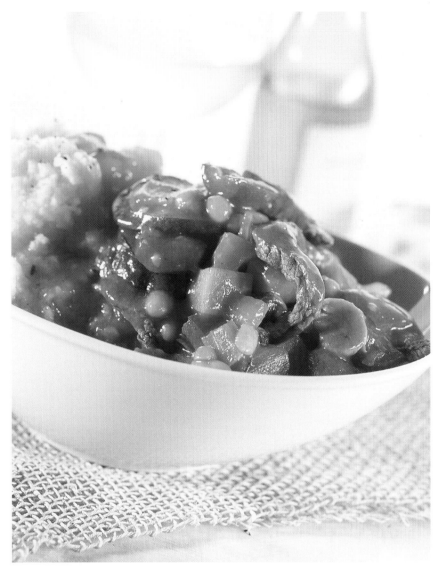

## beef and vegetable hotpot

**1 ¹/₂ tablespooons olive oil**

**1 lb beef strips**

**1 medium yellow onion,
   chopped coarsely**

**1 medium zucchini,
   sliced thickly**

**1 medium sweet red bell pepper,
   coarsely chopped**

**¹/₂ cup coarsely chopped
   orange sweet potato**

**1 trimmed celery stalk,
   chopped coarsely**

**4 oz button mushrooms,
   sliced thickly**

**14 ¹/₂ oz can tomatoes**

**15 oz can baked beans**

Heat oil in pan; cook beef, in batches, until browned. Add onion, stirring until onion is soft. Add zucchini, sweet red bell pepper, orange sweet potato and celery, cook, stirring, 1 minute. Return beef and any juices to pan with mushrooms, undrained crushed tomatoes and baked beans. Bring to boil; simmer, covered, 10 minutes or until vegetables are tender. Serve with mashed potatoes, if desired.

SERVES 4 TO 6

**Storage**  Covered in refrigerator, up to 2 days

**Freeze**  Suitable

☺ FOR BABY  Puree to the desired consistency

☺ FOR TODDLER  Chop appropriately for stage of development

☺ TIP  For a variation, top each serving with a cheesy crouton. Sprinkle grated cheese and chopped parsley onto slices of French bread; broil until cheese melts.

BEEF AND VEGETABLE HOTPOT

## creamy chicken soup

**1 ¹/₂ tablespoons olive oil**

**1 medium yellow onion,
   chopped finely**

**1 clove garlic, crushed**

**4 boneless chicken thighs,
   sliced thinly (1 lb)**

**2 medium carrots,
   chopped coarsely**

**2 trimmed celery stalks,
   chopped coarsely**

**10 oz (1 ¹/₄ cups) canned
   creamed corn**

**4 cups chicken stock**

**1 cup short pasta (shells,
   elbow macaroni, etc)**

**¹/₂ cup cream**

**1 ¹/₂ tablespoons finely chopped
   fresh parsley**

Heat oil in large pan; cook onion and garlic, stirring until onion is soft. Add chicken, carrot, celery, corn and stock, bring to boil; simmer, covered, 20 minutes. Add pasta; simmer uncovered, about 20 minutes or until pasta is tender. Stir in cream; reheat without boiling, sprinkle with parsley to serve.

SERVES 4

**Storage**  Covered in refrigerator, up to 2 days

☺ FOR BABY  Puree to desired consistency

☺ FOR TODDLER  Chop appropriately for stage of development

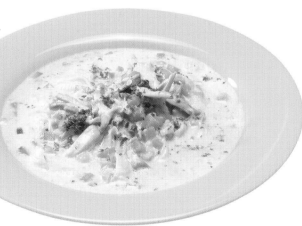

CREAMY CHICKEN SOUP

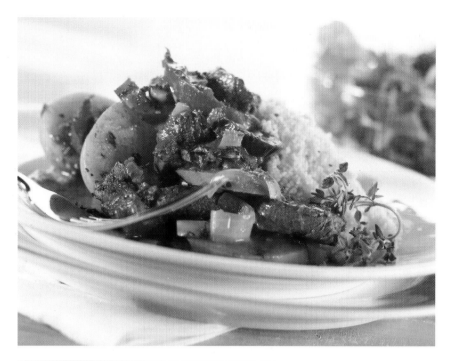

Heat oil in large pan; cook lamb, in batches, until browned all over. Add onion and garlic; cook, stirring, until onion is soft. Return lamb and any juices to pan with potato, carrot, eggplant, sweet red bell pepper, leek, undrained crushed tomatoes, wine (or stock) and herbs; simmer, covered, 1 hour. Add mushrooms; simmer, uncovered, 20 minutes or until lamb is tender and mixture thickens.

SERVES 4

**Storage** Covered, in refrigerator, up to 2 days
**Freeze** Suitable

☺ FOR BABY Puree with cooled boiled water, formula or breast milk to the desired consistency

☺ FOR TODDLER Chop appropriately for stage of development

## home-style chicken casserole

- **2 lb chicken pieces**
- **1 medium yellow onion, sliced thinly**
- **4 oz button mushrooms, halved**
- **2 trimmed celery stalks, sliced thinly**
- **14 1/2 oz can tomatoes**
- **1 clove garlic, crushed**
- **1 teaspoon dried mixed herbs**
- **1 oz envelope French onion soup mix**
- **1 cup dry white wine or water**

Trim excess fat from chicken. Place chicken in greased 14-cup capacity ovenproof dish with onion, mushrooms, celery, undrained crushed tomatoes, garlic and herbs; mix well. Pour combined soup mix and wine (or water) over chicken mixture; bake, uncovered, at 350°F about 1 hour or until chicken is tender. Serve with steamed white rice.

SERVES 4 TO 6

**Storage** Covered, in refrigerator, up to 2 days
**Freeze** Suitable

☺ FOR BABY Remove chicken from bone; puree chicken and sauce with rice to the desired consistency; thin with cooled boiled water, if desired

☺ FOR TODDLER Remove chicken from bone; chop chicken and vegetables appropriately for stage of development; serve with rice, if desired

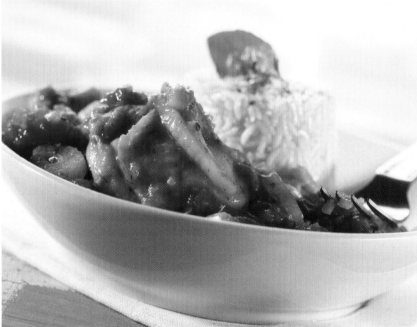

## Mediterranean casserole

*If fresh herbs are unavailable, substitute a half teaspoon each of dried thyme, oregano and basil leaves.*

- **1 1/2 tablespoons olive oil**
- **2 lb diced lamb**
- **1 medium yellow onion, sliced thickly**
- **1 clove garlic, crushed**
- **6 small new potatoes, halved**
- **2 medium carrots, sliced thickly**
- **1 Japanese eggplant, sliced thinly**
- **1 medium sweet red bell pepper, sliced thickly**
- **1 medium leek, sliced thickly**
- **2 x 14 1/2 oz cans tomatoes**
- **1/2 cup dry red wine, or stock**
- **2 teaspoons finely chopped fresh thyme**
- **2 teaspoons finely chopped fresh oregano**
- **2 teaspoons finely chopped fresh basil**
- **4 oz button mushrooms, halved**

## steak and kidney pie

**1 lamb kidney**
**1 lb blade steak, or chuck roast**
**all-purpose flour**
**1 small yellow onion,**
  **chopped finely**
**1 small carrot, chopped coarsely**
**1 trimmed celery stalk,**
  **chopped coarsely**
**1/3 cup coarsely chopped**
  **sweet potato**
**1/2 cup water**
**1/2 cup dry red wine, or extra**
  **water**
**1 unfrozen prepackaged**
  **puff pastry sheet**
**2 teaspoons milk**

Remove skin and fat from kidney; halve lengthwise, remove and discard core of fat. Rinse kidney under cold water; pat dry. Cut kidney into thin slices; cut beef into 3/4-inch cubes. Roll kidney and beef in flour; shake off excess. Combine kidney, beef, vegetables, wine and water in medium pan; bring to boil. Simmer, covered, about 45 minutes or until beef is tender.

Transfer filling mixture to greased 9-inch pie plate; cool 10 minutes. Place pastry over filling; trim to fit dish, brush with milk. Decorate pie with pastry scraps, make 2 small cuts in top; bake at 450°F about 15 minutes or until browned.

SERVES 4 TO 6

**Storage** Covered, in refrigerator, up to 2 days
**Freeze** Cooked filling suitable

☺ FOR BABY Puree filling with cooled boiled water, breast milk or formula to the desired consistency; blend with pureed cooked potato

☺ FOR TODDLER Chop appropriately for stage of development

☺ TIP Instead of pastry, top pie with mashed potatoes sprinkled with combined grated cheese and breadcrumbs.

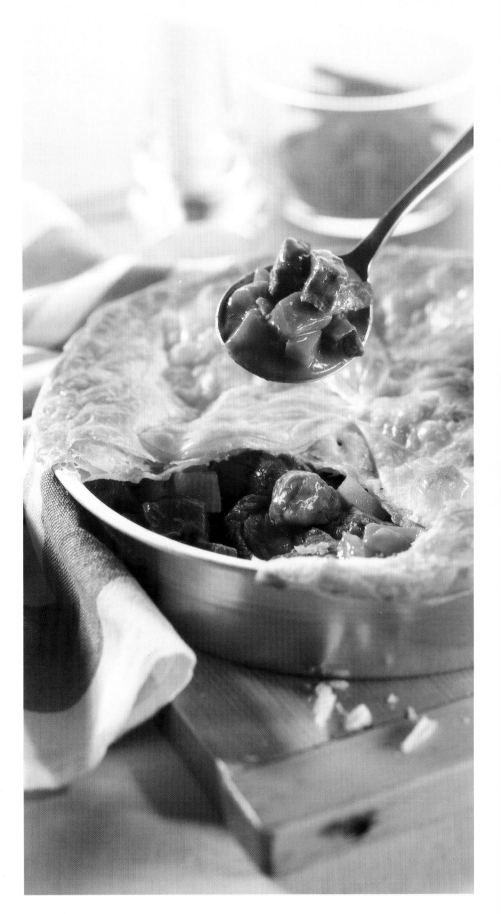

OPPOSITE FROM TOP: MEDITERRANEAN CASSEROLE, HOME-STYLE CHICKEN CASSEROLE
RIGHT: STEAK AND KIDNEY PIE

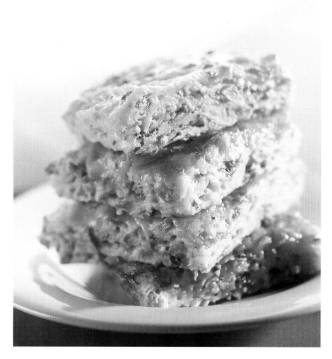
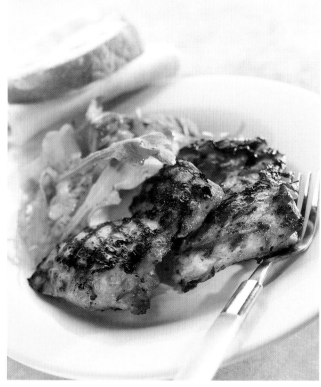

## baked potato, ham and cheese omelette

**4 medium potatoes**
**4 eggs**
**1/2 cup finely chopped ham**
**1 medium tomato,**
**chopped finely**
**2 green onions, chopped finely**
**1 1/2 tablespoons finely chopped**
**fresh parsley**
**1 cup coarsely grated**
**cheddar cheese**

Grate potatoes coarsely; squeeze out excess water. Beat eggs lightly in large bowl; add potato, ham, tomato, onion, parsley and half the cheese, mix well. Spread mixture into greased shallow 6-cup capacity ovenproof dish; sprinkle with remaining cheese. Bake, uncovered, at 350°F about 40 minutes or until browned.

SERVES 4

**Storage** Covered, in refrigerator, up to 2 days

☺ FOR BABY Puree a small quantity with boiled water, formula or breast milk to the desired consistency

☺ FOR TODDLER Serve as above

## glazed thai chicken

**8 boneless chicken thighs (2 1/2 lb)**
**2 teaspoons sweet chili sauce**
**1 teaspoon fish sauce**
**2 teaspoons peanut oil**
**2 teaspoons chopped**
**fresh cilantro**
**1 1/2 tablespoons lime juice**
**2 teaspoons salt-reduced**
**soy sauce**

Trim excess fat from chicken; place chicken in large bowl with remaining ingredients. Cover, refrigerate 2 hours or overnight.

Cook chicken, in batches, on heated oiled griddle (or broiler or barbecue) until browned all over and cooked through. Serve with salad, if desired.

SERVES 4 TO 6

**Storage** Covered, in refrigerator, up to 1 day
**Freeze** Uncooked marinated chicken suitable

☺ FOR BABY Unsuitable

☺ FOR TODDLER Serve as above, finely chopped, with mixed vegetables

## mini burgers

**1 lb ground beef**
**2 teaspoons catsup**
**1 1/2 tablespoons teriyaki sauce**
**1 small yellow onion,**
**chopped finely**
**1 egg**
**6 small brown-and-serve sandwich**
**rolls, or hamburger buns**
**3 tablespoons catsup, extra**
**6 cheese slices**
**2 small plum tomatoes,**
**sliced thinly**
**6 small lettuce leaves**

Combine ground beef, catsup, teriyaki sauce, onion and egg in bowl; shape into 12 patties. (Freeze 6 patties for later use.)

Cook patties on heated oiled griddle or skillet until cooked through.

Meanwhile, bake rolls according to manufacturer's instructions; split in half. Spread bottoms with extra catsup; top with patties then cheese. Broil until cheese melts; top with tomato, lettuce and remaining half of roll.

MAKES 6

*Best assembled just before serving*

**Freeze** Uncooked patties suitable

☺ FOR BABY Puree patties with cooled boiled water to the desired consistency

☺ FOR TODDLER Serve quartered

*ABOVE FROM LEFT: BAKED POTATO, HAM AND CHEESE OMELETTE; GLAZED THAI CHICKEN*

# bright ideas for barbecuing

Toddlers love a family barbecue as much as everyone else and let's be honest — a 2-year-old with a burger is considerably less worrying on the back lawn than on the dining room carpet!

• When adapting barbecue recipes for toddlers, reserve small portions of meat and flavor with simple marinades, such as salt-reduced soy sauce or honey. Thread onto bamboo skewers to cook (with fruit or veggies, if desired) but make sure skewer is removed before serving. For smaller babies, barbecued meat can be pureed or chopped finely.

• Toddlers also love chops, chicken drumsticks and small ears of corn.

• Serve simple, accessible salads — lettuce, cherry tomatoes, blanched vegetable sticks, chunks of cheese, hard-boiled eggs or barbecued vegetables. Toddlers will happily pick their favorites.

• Food wrapped in bread is an easy way for a toddler to manage food outdoors. Avoid giving them big rolls, or bread that is too thick — both are awkward to hold and eat. Try tortillas, Lebanese or pita bread filled with small pieces of meat and salad. Mini-burgers and small steak sandwiches are also popular with toddlers.

• Sausages wrapped in fresh, buttered bread with catsup (choose salt-reduced) are perennial favorites with toddlers and adults alike. For a change, try sausages wrapped in cracker bread with hummus. Smaller tots can have finely chopped skinless sausage alone or with their vegetables.

*MINI BURGERS*

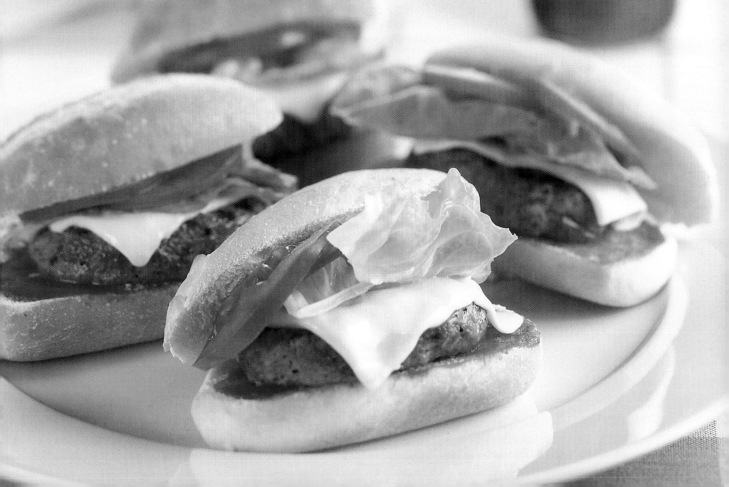

## winter squash and orange sweet potato soup

**1 1/2 tablespoons olive oil**
**1 medium yellow onion, chopped**
**2 teaspoons finely grated**
**fresh ginger**
**1 green banana pepper,**
**seeded, chopped**
**1 1/2 tablespoons finely chopped**
**fresh lemon grass**
**2 teaspoons ground cumin**
**2 teaspoons ground coriander**
**1 teaspoon ground turmeric**
**1 lb trimmed winter squash,**
**chopped coarsely**
**1 lb orange sweet potato,**
**chopped coarsely**
**6 cups chicken stock**
**1/4 cup coconut cream**

Heat oil; cook onion until soft. Add ginger, pepper, lemon grass and spices; cook, stirring, until fragrant. Add winter squash and sweet potato; cook, stirring, 1 minute. Add stock, bring to boil; simmer, covered about 20 minutes or until vegetables are tender. Cool 10 minutes; blend or process, in batches, until smooth.

Serve in individual serving bowls, swirl with coconut cream; top with croutons, if desired.

SERVES 4 TO 6

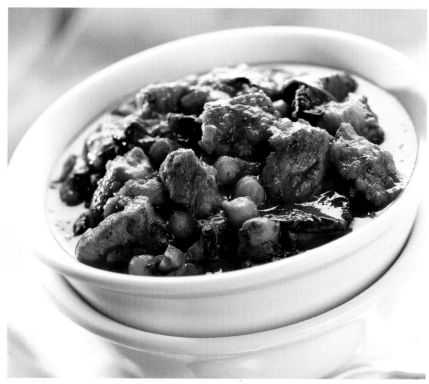

PORK AND GARBANZO CURRY

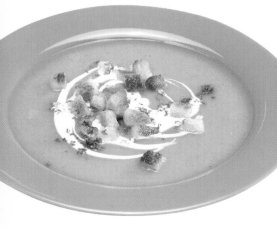

WINTER SQUASH AND
ORANGE SWEET POTATO SOUP

**Storage** Covered, in refrigerator, up to 2 days
**Freeze** Suitable

☺ FOR BABY Puree with cooled boiled water to the desired consistency; serve without croutons

☺ FOR TODDLER Serve as above

## pork and garbanzo curry

**1 lb boneless pork chops**
**1 large yellow onion, sliced thinly**
**1 1/2 tablespoons mild curry paste**
**14 1/2 oz can tomatoes**
**3/4 cup vegetable stock**
**8 3/4 oz can garbanzos, rinsed, drained**
**1/2 cup coconut milk**
**10 1/2 oz spinach, trimmed**
**2 teaspoons chopped fresh cilantro**

Cut pork into 3/4-inch cubes; cook, uncovered, in large heated oiled pan, in batches, until well browned. Add onion and paste; cook, uncovered, until onion is soft. Return pork to pan; stir in undrained crushed tomatoes and stock. Bring to boil; simmer, covered, 45 minutes. Stir in garbanzos, bring to boil; simmer, uncovered, stirring occasionally, about 15 minutes or until garbanzos are tender. Stir in milk, spinach and cilantro; cook, stirring, until spinach is just wilted.

SERVES 4

**Storage** Covered, in refrigerator, up to 2 days
**Freeze** Suitable before adding coconut milk, spinach and cilantro

☺ FOR BABY Unsuitable

☺ FOR TODDLER Serve as above, chopped finely

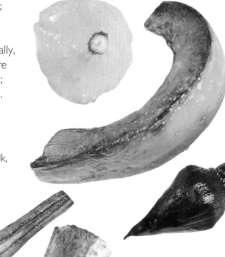

## roast rib-eye steak with garlic rosemary potatoes

**3 lb rib-eye steak**

**1 1/2 tablespoons olive oil**

**2 teaspoons cracked black pepper**

**6 medium potatoes, quartered (2 lb)**

**2 cloves garlic, crushed**

**1 1/2 tablespoons fresh rosemary**

**3 tablespoons olive oil, extra**

Place beef on wire rack in baking dish, rub with oil then pepper; bake, uncovered, at 450°F 15 minutes. Remove from oven, reduce heat to 350°F. Add combined potatoes, garlic, rosemary and extra oil to dish; bake, uncovered, about 45 minutes or until cooked as desired. Serve with stoneground mustard and seasonal vegetables.

SERVES 4 TO 6

*Best made just before serving*

☺ FOR BABY  Select beef without pepper, puree beef and vegetables with breast milk, formula or cooled boiled water to the desired consistency

☺ FOR TODDLER  Select beef without pepper, chop beef and vegetables appropriately for stage of development

☺ TIP  There is nothing better to tempt toddlers to eat their veggies than mixed roast vegetables. Use as wide a variety as possible to help introduce new flavors.

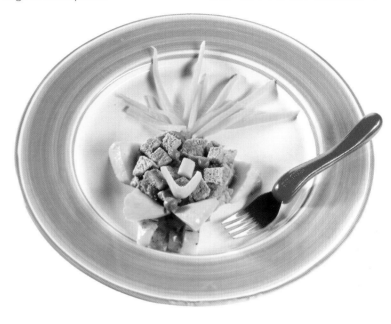

ROAST RIB-EYE STEAK WITH GARLIC ROSEMARY POTATOES, TODDLER SERVING

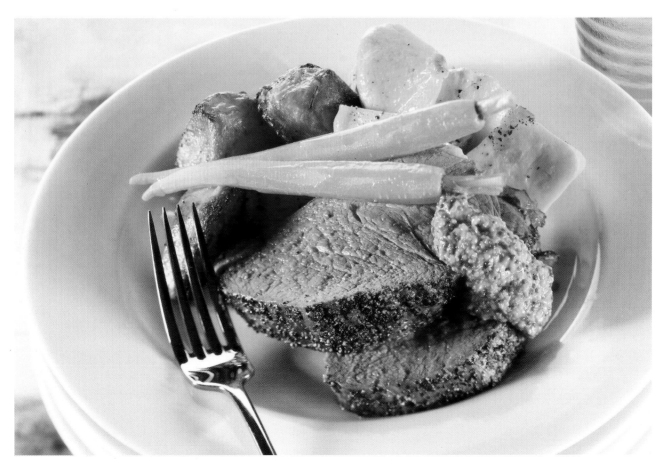

ROAST RIB-EYE STEAK WITH GARLIC ROSEMARY POTATOES

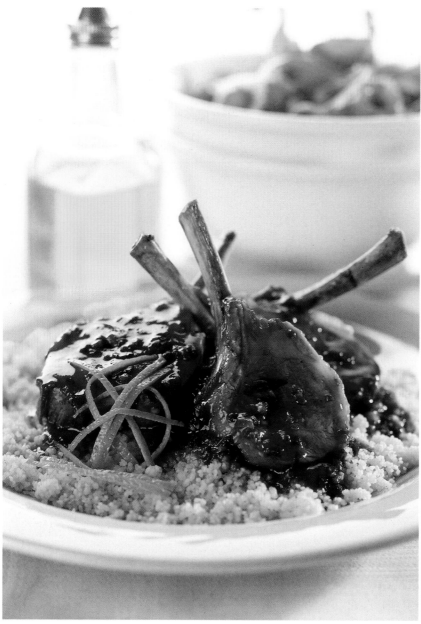

RACK OF LAMB WITH ORANGE COUSCOUS

## rack of lamb with orange
### COUSCOUS

**2 racks of lamb with
8 ribs each**
**¹/2 cup orange juice**
**¹/4 cup red currant jelly**
**¹/4 cup dry white wine or stock**
**3 tablespoons finely chopped
fresh chives**

ORANGE COUSCOUS
**1 ¹/3 cups orange juice**
**2 cloves**
**1 bay leaf**
**¹/2 teaspoon ground cinnamon**
**1 ¹/2 cups couscous**
**2 tablespoons butter**

Place lamb on wire rack in baking dish; bake, uncovered, at 400°F 35 minutes or until cooked as desired.

Meanwhile, combine juice, jelly, wine (or stock) and chives in small pan; simmer, uncovered, until thickened slightly. Serve lamb with sauce and Orange Couscous.

**Orange Couscous** Combine juice, cloves, bay leaf and cinnamon in medium pan, bring to boil; remove from heat. Stir in couscous; let stand 3 minutes or until liquid is absorbed. Stir in chopped butter; discard cloves and bay leaf before serving.

SERVES 4

*Best made just before serving*

☺ FOR BABY  Remove lamb from bone; puree lamb and couscous with cooled boiled water to the desired consistency

☺ FOR TODDLER  Remove lamb from bone; chop to suit appropriate stage of development, serve with couscous

## lamb drumsticks

*French-trimmed lamb shanks are called "drumsticks" by some butchers, the shanks having been trimmed of all sinew and fat so they resemble a gigantic chicken leg.*

**6 lamb "drumsticks"**
**¹/2 cup honey**
**¹/4 cup soy sauce**
**1 teaspoon Dijon mustard**

Make diagonal cuts, about 3/8 inch apart, through to bone on both sides of shanks. Place in greased shallow ovenproof dish; pour over combined remaining ingredients. Cover, refrigerate 2 hours or overnight.

Bake, uncovered, at 350°F about 40 minutes or until tender, brushing twice during cooking with pan juices. Serve with cooked pasta and carrots, if desired.

SERVES 6

**Storage**  Covered, in refrigerator, up to 2 days
**Freeze**  Uncooked marinated lamb suitable

☺ FOR BABY  Remove lamb from bone; puree lamb, pasta and carrots with cooled boiled water to the desired consistency

☺ FOR TODDLER  Trim lamb drumstick appropriately for stage of development; serve with pasta and carrots

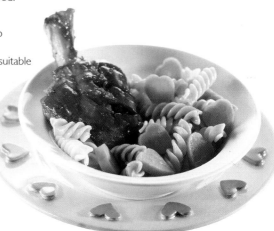

LAMB DRUMSTICKS, TODDLER SERVING

## sunday roast

**3 lb chicken**

**1 medium onion,
    sliced thickly**

**1 medium lemon,
    sliced thickly**

**2 teaspoons olive oil**

**1 teaspoon salt**

**4 medium potatoes, halved**

**2 lb pumpkin, or winter squash,
    cut into chunks**

**2 medium onions,
    halved, extra**

**2 medium tomatoes, halved**

MUSHROOM GRAVY

**3¹/₂ oz button mushrooms,
    sliced thinly**

**1¹/₂ tablespoons all-purpose flour**

**¹/₂ cup chicken stock**

**¹/₂ cup white wine (or extra
    stock, if preferred)**

Wash chicken thoroughly; dry with paper towels. Place sliced onion and lemon inside cavity; secure opening with toothpick or skewer. Tie legs of chicken together with kitchen string; tuck wings under. Rub oil and salt all over chicken.

Place chicken, breast-side up, with potatoes, pumpkin or winter squash and onion halves in oiled flameproof baking dish. Cover chicken with oiled foil; bake at 350°F 45 minutes. Remove foil, add tomatoes; bake about 45 minutes or until chicken is cooked through and vegetables are tender. Serve with Mushroom Gravy.

**Mushroom Gravy** Transfer chicken and vegetables to serving dish. Cover to keep warm. Reserve 3 tablespoons of the pan juices, discarding extra fat. Heat juices and mushrooms in baking dish; stir in flour.

Cook, stirring, until mixture is well browned; gradually stir in combined stock and wine (if using). Bring to boil; simmer, stirring, about 5 minutes or until gravy boils and thickens.

SERVES 4

*Best made just before serving*

☺ FOR BABY Puree chicken and vegetables separately with cooled boiled water to the desired consistency. Stir through a little gravy, if desired

☺ FOR TODDLER Remove chicken from bone; chop appropriately for stage of development, serve with accompaniments

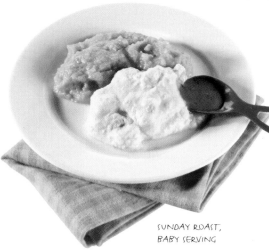

SUNDAY ROAST,
BABY SERVING

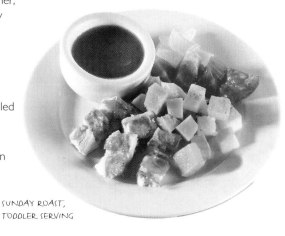

SUNDAY ROAST,
TODDLER SERVING

SUNDAY ROAST

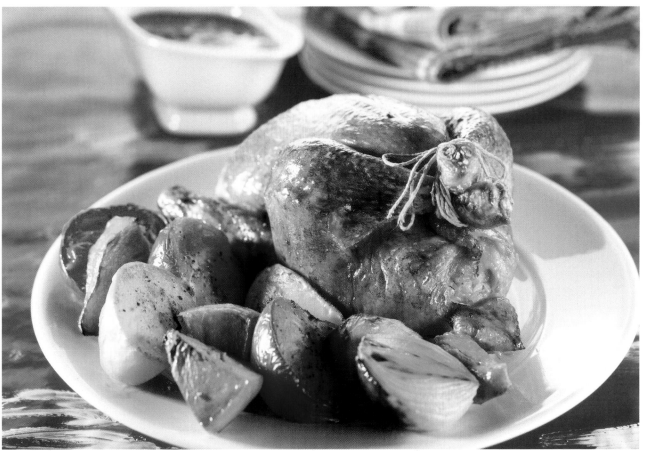

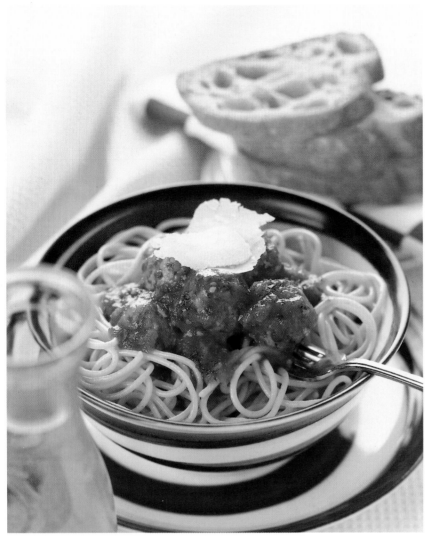

ITALIAN MEATBALLS IN TOMATO BASIL SAUCE

**Storage** Cover cooked Meatballs and Tomato Basil Sauce, separately; refrigerate up to 2 days

**Freeze** Uncooked meatballs suitable

☺ FOR BABY Puree small quantities of pasta and sauce with 1 meatball to the desired consistency

☺ FOR TODDLER Chop meatballs and spaghetti appropriately for stage of development

## cheese souffle

**3 tablespoons packaged breadcrumbs**
**1/4 cup butter**
**1/4 cup all-purpose flour**
**1 cup milk**
**1 cup coarsely grated cheddar cheese**
**3 eggs, separated**

Grease four 1-cup ovenproof dishes; sprinkle bottoms and sides with breadcrumbs, place on baking sheet.

Melt butter in medium pan, add flour; cook, stirring, until mixture thickens and bubbles. Gradually stir in milk; stir until mixture boils and thickens. Remove from heat; let stand 2 minutes, stir in cheese and egg yolks. Transfer mixture to large bowl, cover surface with plastic wrap; cool.

Beat egg whites in medium bowl with electric mixer until firm peaks form. Fold about a third of the egg whites into souffle mixture then fold in remainder. Divide mixture among prepared dishes; bake at 450°F about 20 minutes or until puffed and browned.

SERVES 4

*Best made just before serving*

☺ FOR BABY Puree to the desired consistency

☺ FOR TODDLER Serve as above, with salad, if desired

CHEESE SOUFFLE

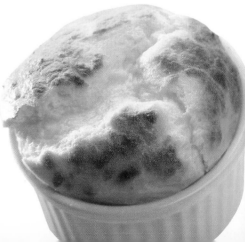

## Italian meatballs in tomato basil sauce

*If fresh herbs are unavailable, substitute half a teaspoon each dried basil and mint.*

**1/2 lb ground pork**
**1/2 lb ground veal**
**1 medium zucchini, grated coarsely**
**1 medium onion, chopped finely**
**1 egg, beaten lightly**
**1/2 cup fresh breadcrumbs**
**1/4 cup catsup**
**1 1/2 tablespoons finely chopped fresh basil**
**1 1/2 tablespoons finely chopped fresh mint**
**1 lb spaghetti**
**1/3 cup shaved parmesan cheese**

TOMATO BASIL SAUCE
**14 oz can tomatoes**
**15 oz can tomato puree**
**2 cloves garlic, crushed**
**1/4 cup finely chopped fresh basil**
**1 teaspoon sugar**

Combine ground meats, zucchini, onion, egg, breadcrumbs, catsup and herbs in medium bowl; mix well. Roll rounded tablespoons of mixture into balls. Place on oiled foil-lined baking sheet; bake at 400°F 25 minutes.

Meanwhile, cook spaghetti in large pot of boiling water, uncovered, until just tender; drain. Toss meatballs through sauce; serve over hot spaghetti and sprinkle with parmesan cheese.

**Tomato Basil Sauce** Combine undrained crushed tomatoes, puree, garlic, basil and sugar in medium pan; simmer, uncovered, about 15 minutes or until thickened.

## pasta Siciliana

*We used penne in this recipe but you can use any short pasta.*

**3 tablespoons olive oil**
**1 medium onion, chopped finely**
**1 clove garlic, crushed**
**2 medium zucchini, chopped coarsely**
**2 Japanese eggplants, sliced thickly**
**2 medium tomatoes, peeled, chopped**
**1 medium green bell pepper, sliced thinly**
**15 oz can tomato puree**
**1/2 cup dry red wine (or stock)**
**1/4 teaspoon brown sugar**
**1 lb pasta**
**3 tablespoons finely chopped fresh basil**
**1/2 cup finely grated parmesan cheese**

Heat oil in large pan; cook onion and garlic, stirring, until onion is soft. Add zucchini, eggplant, tomato and bell pepper; cook, stirring, until vegetables are tender. Stir in puree, wine (or stock) and sugar; simmer, uncovered, 5 minutes or until mixture thickens slightly.

Meanwhile, cook pasta in large pot of boiling water, uncovered, until just tender; drain. Toss sauce through pasta; sprinkle basil and cheese over pasta just before serving.

SERVES 4 TO 6

**Storage** Vegetable mixture, covered, in refrigerator up to 2 days

☺ FOR BABY Puree pasta and sauce (without basil and cheese) with cooled boiled water to the desired consistency

☺ FOR TODDLER Chop appropriately for stage of development

BAKED FAVA BEAN AND LEEK PASTA

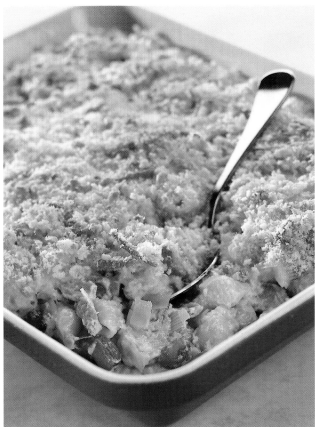

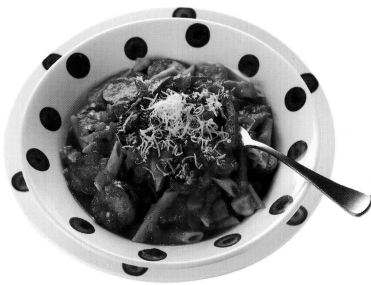

PASTA SICILIANA

## baked fava bean and leek pasta

**1 cup short pasta (shells, elbow macaroni, etc.)**
**1 lb packet frozen fava beans**
**1/2 cup butter**
**1 large leek, chopped coarsely**
**1/4 cup all-purpose flour**
**1 quart milk**
**3/4 cup coarsely grated cheddar cheese**
**3 x 6 oz cans tuna, drained, flaked**
**1 cup fresh breadcrumbs**

Cook pasta in large pot of boiling water, uncovered, until just tender; drain.

Boil, steam or microwave fava beans until tender; drain. Refresh under cold water; then remove and discard outer skins. Melt half of the butter in large pan; cook leek, stirring, until tender. Combine leek mixture in large bowl with pasta and fava beans.

Melt remaining butter in medium pan, add flour; cook, stirring, until mixture thickens and bubbles. Gradually stir in milk; stir until mixture boils and thickens, stir in half of the cheese. Combine cheese sauce and tuna in bowl with pasta and vegetables; mix well. Spoon pasta mixture into oiled 12-cup capacity ovenproof dish; sprinkle with combined breadcrumbs and remaining cheese. Bake, uncovered, at 350°F about 20 minutes or until heated through and browned lightly.

SERVES 4 TO 6

**Storage** Covered, in refrigerator, up to 2 days
**Freeze** Suitable

☺ FOR BABY Puree with cooled boiled water to the desired consistency

☺ FOR TODDLER Chop appropriately for stage of development

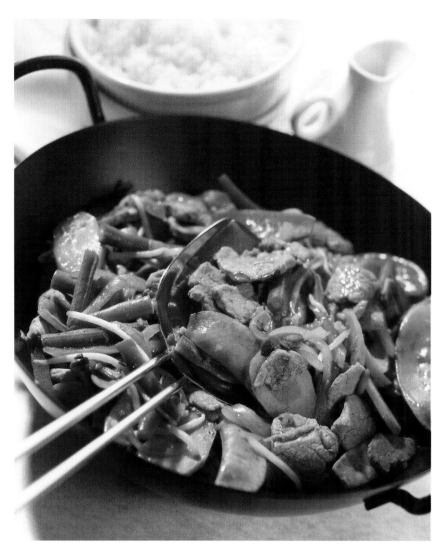

## pork and vegetable stir-fry

**3 tablespoons vegetable oil**
**1 lb boneless pork chops,**
  **sliced thinly**
**1 medium onion, sliced thinly**
**1 clove garlic, crushed**
**1 medium carrot,**
  **sliced thinly**
**4 oz mushrooms, sliced thinly**
**5 oz green beans, halved**
**5 oz snow peas**
**1 cup bean sprouts**
**3 tablespoons oyster sauce**
**1 1/2 tablespoons plum sauce**
**1 1/2 tablespoons sherry or stock**

Heat half the oil in wok or large pan; stir-fry pork, in batches, until browned all over. Heat remaining oil in wok; stir-fry onion and garlic 1 minute. Add carrot, mushroom, and beans; stir-fry until vegetables are just tender. Return pork to pan with snow peas, sprouts, sauces and sherry or stock; stir-fry until hot. Serve with steamed jasmine rice, if desired.

SERVES 4 TO 6

*Best made just before serving*

🙂 FOR BABY  Unsuitable

🙂 FOR TODDLER  Chop appropriately for stage of development

*LEFT: PORK AND VEGETABLE STIR-FRY*
*BELOW: VEGETABLE LASAGNE*

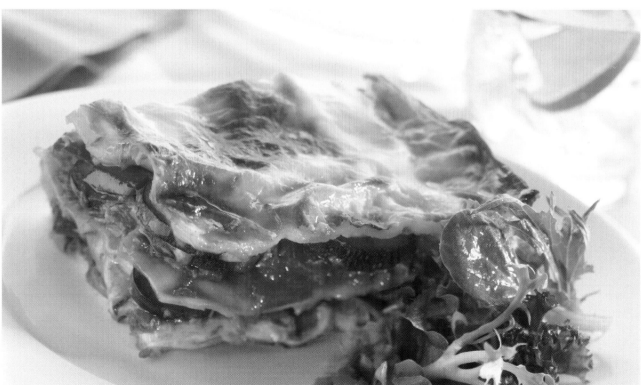

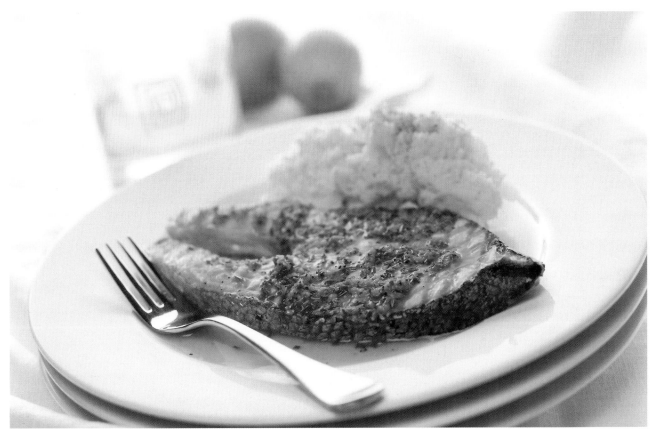

ATLANTIC SALMON WITH CITRUS BUTTER SAUCE

## vegetable lasagna

**1 1/2 tablespoons olive oil**
**1 medium onion,**
  **chopped finely**
**1 clove garlic, crushed**
**2 medium sweet red bell**
  **peppers, chopped coarsely**
**2 medium zucchini,**
  **sliced thinly**
**2 Japanese eggplants,**
  **sliced thinly**
**2 oz mushrooms, sliced thinly**
**3 tablespoons tomato paste**
**14 oz can tomatoes**
**1/2 cup dry white wine or stock**
**8 oz cooked lasagna sheets**
**1/3 cup finely grated parmesan**
  **cheese**

WHITE SAUCE
**1/4 cup butter**
**1/4 cup all-purpose flour**
**2 cups milk**
**1/2 cup grated cheddar**
  **cheese**

Heat oil in large pan; cook onion and garlic, stirring, until onion is soft. Add bell pepper, zucchini and eggplant; cook, stirring, until vegetables have softened. Stir in mushrooms, tomato paste, undrained crushed tomatoes and wine or stock; simmer, uncovered, about 15 minutes or until mixture thickens slightly.

Place one layer of cooked lasagna noodles over bottom of greased 2-quart ovenproof dish. Top with half the vegetable mixture and a third of the White Sauce. Repeat layering in this way, finishing with a layer of lasagna noodles. Pour remaining White Sauce over lasagna; sprinkle with cheese. Bake, uncovered, at 350°F about 40 minutes or until browned lightly and heated through. Serve with green salad, if desired.

**White Sauce** Melt butter in medium pan, add flour; cook, stirring, until mixture thickens and bubbles. Gradually add milk, stirring, until mixture boils and thickens; stir in cheese.

SERVES 4 TO 6

**Storage** Covered, in refrigerator, up to 2 days
**Freeze** Suitable

☺ FOR BABY Puree with cooled boiled water to the desired consistency

☺ FOR TODDLER Chop appropriately for stage of development

## Atlantic salmon with citrus butter sauce

*Lime rind and juice can be substituted for lemon in this recipe.*

**4 salmon steaks (about 2 lb)**
**1/4 cup butter**
**2 teaspoons finely grated**
  **lemon rind**
**3 tablespoons lemon juice**
**1 1/2 tablespoons finely chopped**
  **fresh chives**
**1/2 teaspoon cracked**
  **black pepper**

Cook salmon on heated oiled griddle (or broiler or barbecue) until browned and cooked as desired; cover to keep warm. Combine remaining ingredients in small pan; cook, stirring, until butter is melted. Serve salmon drizzled with citrus butter sauce and mashed potato, if desired.

SERVES 4

*Best made just before serving*

☺ FOR BABY Omit pepper; puree salmon with cooled boiled water, and mashed potato if desired, to the desired consistency

☺ FOR TODDLER Omit pepper; chop salmon appropriately for stage of development, serve with mashed potato

## baked orange cheesecake

**7 oz sugar cookies**

**1/2 cup butter, melted**

**2 eggs**

**1/3 cup sugar**

**8 oz packaged cream cheese**

**8 oz ricotta cheese**

**1 1/2 tablespoons orange rind,
    finely grated**

**3 tablespoons orange juice**

Line bottom of 8-inch round springform pan with foil, grease bottom and side.

Process cookies until crushed finely; add butter, process until just combined. Press cookie mixture evenly over bottom and side of prepared pan, leaving 1-inch border. Cover; refrigerate 1 hour.

Beat eggs and sugar in medium bowl with electric mixer until thick and creamy; add cheeses, rind and juice, beat cheese mixture until smooth.

Place springform pan on baking sheet; pour cheese mixture into pan. Bake at 350°F about 1 hour or until firm. Cool in oven with door ajar. Cover cheesecake; refrigerate 3 hours or overnight. Serve with orange segments, if desired.

SERVES 4 TO 6

**Storage** Refrigerate, covered, up to 3 days

☺ FOR BABY Older babies can eat filling if it is finely sieved

☺ FOR TODDLER Serve as above

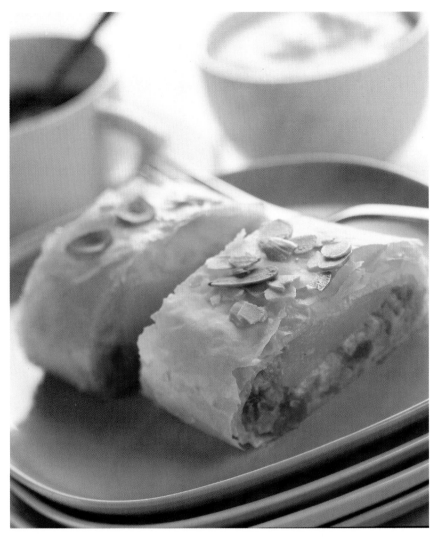

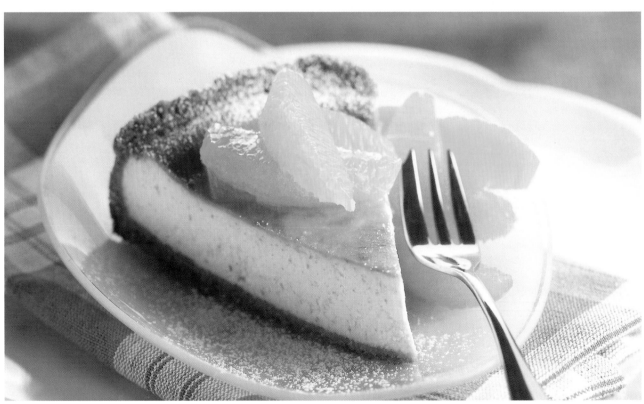

## citrus delicious

**3 eggs, separated**
**1/2 cup superfine sugar**
**1/2 cup self-rising flour**
**2 tablespoons butter, melted**
**1 cup milk**
**1 teaspoon grated orange rind**
**1 teaspoon grated lemon rind**
**1/3 cup lemon juice**
**1/2 cup superfine sugar, extra**

Grease four 1-cup capacity ovenproof dishes.

Beat egg yolks and sugar in medium bowl with electric mixer until thick and creamy; stir in sifted flour then butter, milk, rind, and juice.

Beat egg whites in small bowl with electric mixer until soft peaks form; gradually add extra sugar, beat until dissolved. Fold egg white mixture, in 2 batches, into lemon mixture; divide mixture among prepared dishes. Place dishes in large baking dish with enough boiling water to come halfway up sides; bake at 350°F about 20 minutes or until set. Dust with powdered sugar to serve, if desired.

SERVES 4

*Best made just before serving*

☺ FOR BABY  Puree to the desired consistency

☺ FOR TODDLER  Serve as above

## pear and ricotta strudel

**6 sheets filo pastry**
**3 1/2 tablespoons butter, melted**
**15 oz can pear halves, drained, sliced thickly**
**1 1/2 tablespoons flaked almonds**

RICOTTA FILLING
**1 cup ricotta cheese**
**1/3 cup fresh breadcrumbs**
**1/4 cup finely chopped dried apricots**
**3 tablespoons finely chopped almonds, toasted**
**1/4 cup powdered sugar**
**1/2 teaspoon ground cinnamon**

Brush each filo sheet with butter; layer sheets on top of each other on buttered baking sheet.

Spread filling 1 inch from edge of 1 long side and 2 1/2 inches from both ends; top with pears. Roll pastry to enclose filling, tucking in ends; position seam-side

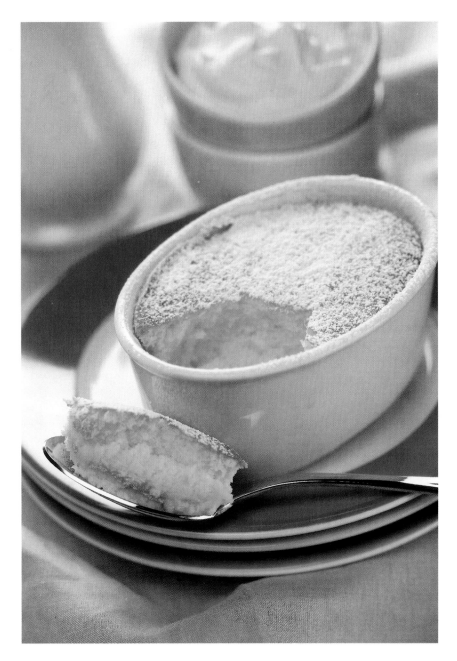

down, brush all over with remaining butter. Sprinkle with almonds; bake at 350°F about 25 minutes or until browned lightly. Serve with cream, if desired.

**Ricotta Filling**  Combine all ingredients in medium bowl; mix well.

SERVES 4

*Best made just before serving*

☺ FOR BABY  Omit almonds; puree cooked filling mixture with cooled boiled water, breast milk or formula to the desired consistency

☺ FOR TODDLER  Omit almonds; serve as above, with ice cream, if desired

*OPPOSITE FROM TOP: PEAR AND RICOTTA STRUDEL; BAKED ORANGE CHEESECAKE ABOVE: CITRUS DELICIOUS*

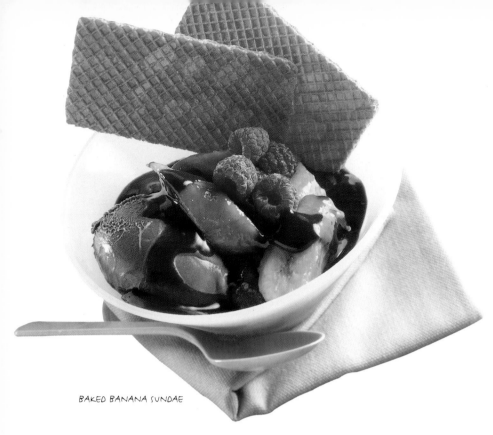

BAKED BANANA SUNDAE

## rhubarb and berry compote

**1/2 cup superfine sugar**
**1 cup water**
**3 tablespoons lemon juice**
**3 cups coarsely chopped fresh rhubarb**
**8 oz strawberries, quartered**
**1 cup blueberries**

Combine sugar, water and juice in medium pan; stir over heat, without boiling, until sugar dissolves. Add rhubarb; simmer, covered, 2 minutes or until just tender. Transfer to large bowl, stir in strawberries and blueberries; cool. Serve with cream, if desired.

SERVES 4 TO 6

**Storage**  Covered, in refrigerator, up to 2 days

☺ FOR BABY  Puree rhubarb to the desired consistency; stir through blended cereal, if desired

☺ FOR TODDLER  Serve a small portion with cream or custard

## baked banana sundae

**1/4 cup butter**
**1/3 cup firmly packed brown sugar**
**8 small bananas**
**1 quart chocolate ice cream**
**5 oz fresh raspberries**
**8 wafer cookies**

CHOCOLATE FUDGE SAUCE
**1/2 cup cream**
**1/4 cup superfine sugar**
**4 oz dark chocolate, chopped finely**
**1 teaspoon vanilla extract**

Heat butter in large heavy-bottomed pan; cook sugar, stirring, until dissolved. Add bananas; cook, turning occasionally, until just tender. Serve warm bananas with ice cream, raspberries, wafers and Chocolate Fudge Sauce.

**Chocolate Fudge Sauce**  Combine cream and sugar in small pan; cook over very low heat, stirring, until sugar is dissolved. Remove pan from heat; add chocolate and vanilla, stirring until chocolate melts. Serve sauce warm or cold.

SERVES 4 TO 6

**Storage**  Chocolate Fudge Sauce can be made up to a week ahead; keep, covered, in refrigerator

☺ FOR BABY  Puree cooked bananas to the desired consistency

☺ FOR TODDLERS  Serve as above

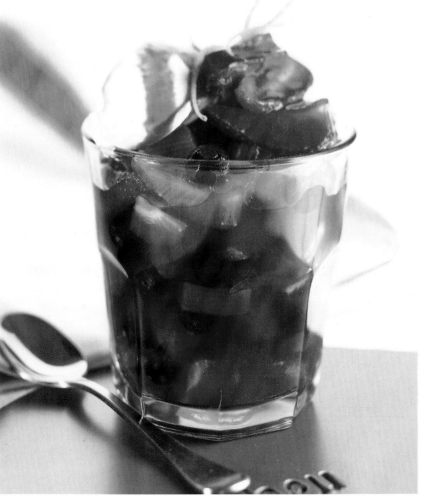

RHUBARB AND BERRY COMPOTE

## chocolate mousse

**4 oz dark chocolate patties**
**1 1/2 tablespoons orange juice**
**4 eggs, separated**
**1 1/2 cups thickened cream**

Stir chocolate, in small heatproof bowl over pan of simmering water, until melted, remove from heat; cool. Stir in juice then egg yolks; fold cream into chocolate mixture; transfer mixture to large bowl.

Beat egg whites in small bowl with electric mixer until soft peaks form. Fold egg whites into chocolate cream mixture, in 2 batches. Spoon mixture into serving dishes, cover; refrigerate 3 hours or overnight. Dust with cocoa and serve with strawberries, if desired.

SERVES 4 TO 6

*Best made a day ahead*

Storage  Covered, in refrigerator, up to 2 days

☺ FOR BABY  Unsuitable

☺ FOR TODDLER  Serve as above

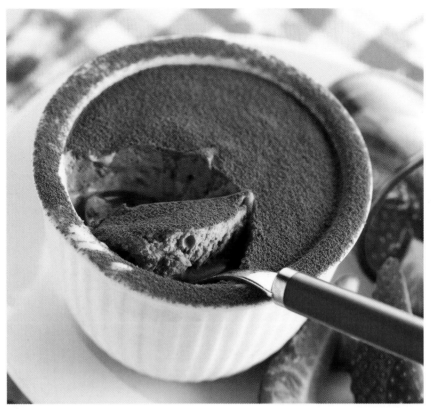

CHOCOLATE MOUSSE

## saucy butterscotch pudding

**1 cup self-rising flour**
**1/2 cup ground almonds**
**1/2 cup firmly packed brown sugar**
**2/3 cup milk**
**1/4 cup butter, melted**
**1 egg, beaten lightly**

BUTTERSCOTCH SAUCE
**1/2 cup water**
**1 cup cream**
**1/2 cup golden syrup, maple syrup or Karo syrup**
**3 tablespoons butter**

Grease 2-quart ovenproof dish. Sift combined flour, ground almonds and sugar into large bowl; add combined milk, butter and egg, stir until smooth. Pour mixture into prepared dish; pour hot Butterscotch Sauce carefully over pudding. Bake at 350°F about 35 minutes or until pudding is firm. Serve with whipped cream, if desired.

Butterscotch Sauce  Combine all ingredients in medium pan; cook, stirring, without boiling, about 2 minutes or until butter has melted.

SERVES 4

*Best made just before serving*

☺ FOR BABY  Unsuitable

☺ FOR TODDLER  Serve as above, with ice cream, if desired.

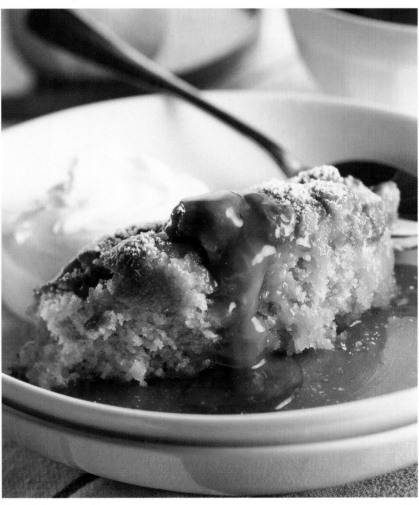

SAUCY BUTTERSCOTCH PUDDING

# party food and birthday cakes

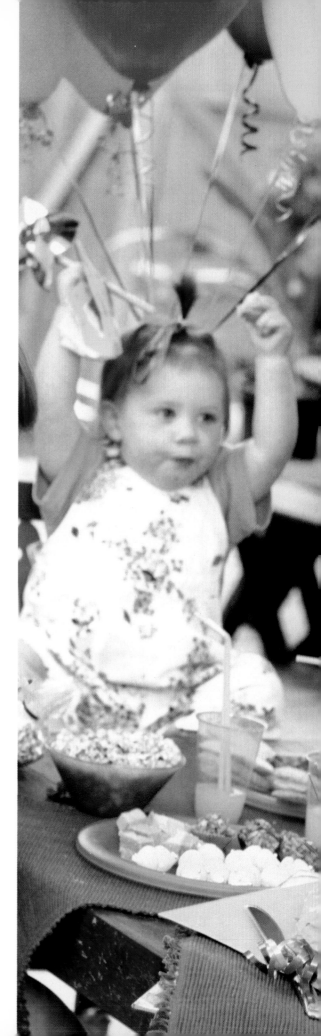

Although no one would argue that healthy food is best, when birthdays and parties come around it is wise to accept from the outset that the five food groups may take somewhat of a battering. You do not have to turn the affair into one giant sugar fest either, but there is no need to panic at occasional over-indulgence. Children quickly learn to value a special celebration as much as we do and if "party food" is only associated with parties, then it is not going to interfere too much with everyday routine. Bear in mind as well that little ones are usually so excited by the fun of a party, they actually do not eat a great deal. Anyone who has ever cleaned up after a small child's party knows that birthday cake is usually mashed around the plate and left – it is the candles and singing that form the unforgettable part of the experience. Only the adults ever seem to remember what flavor the cake was!

So do not get upset making traffic-light sandwiches with tomato and cheese – no one has ever met a child who would eat one of these. On the other hand, there *are* ways of making party food slightly less unhealthy, without making it seem any less special or delicious and on the following pages you will find lots of recipes and ideas. Do not think for a minute that you need to make *everything*. Choose one or two sweet things and a couple of salty ones – and have fun!

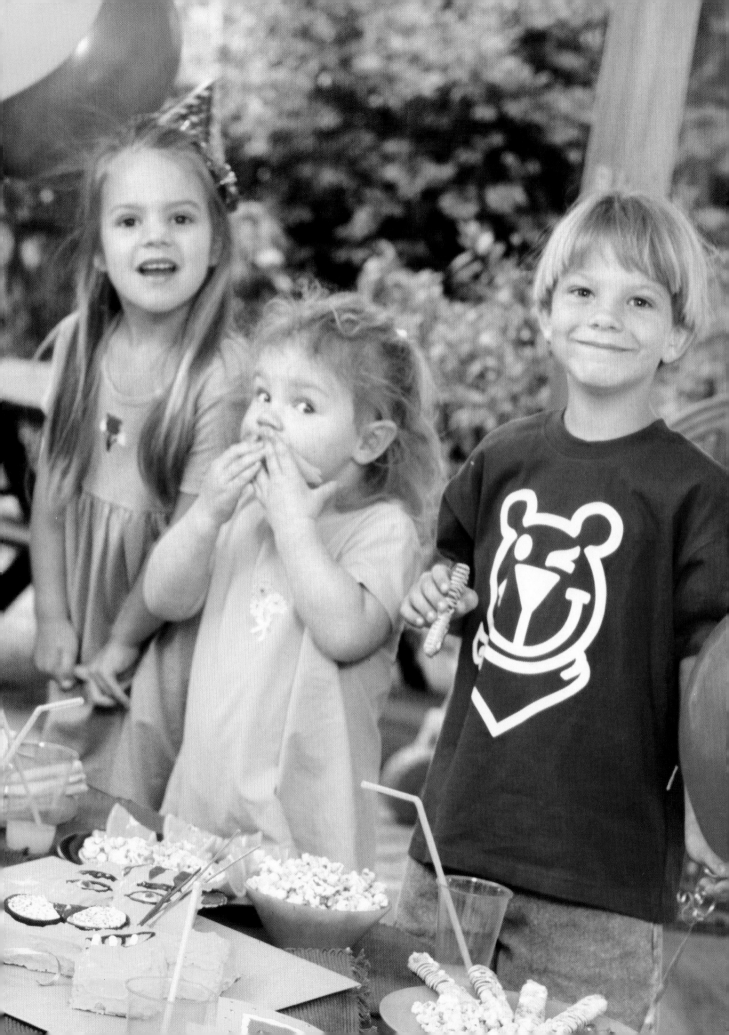

## noodle pancakes

*Pancakes may be served hot or at room temperature. We used rice noodles in this batter.*

**2 oz rice noodles**
**1/4 cup all-purpose flour**
**1 green onion, sliced finely**
**1 clove garlic, crushed**
**1 teaspoon grated fresh ginger**
**1/2 teaspoon ground coriander**
**3 tablespoons coconut milk**
**peanut oil, for frying**

Place noodles in small heatproof bowl, cover with boiling water, let stand until just tender; drain. Cut noodles into 2-inch lengths; combine in medium bowl with flour, onion, garlic, ginger, coriander and milk. Heat oil in large pan; fry rounded tablespoons of mixture, in batches, until browned both sides and cooked through. Drain on paper towels; serve with plum or sweet and sour sauce, if desired.

MAKES 12

**Storage** Best made just before serving

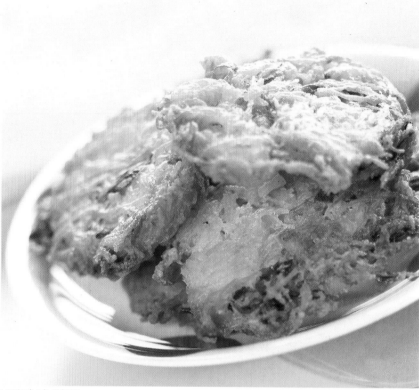

NOODLE PANCAKES

CHICKEN NUGGETS WITH OVEN FRIES

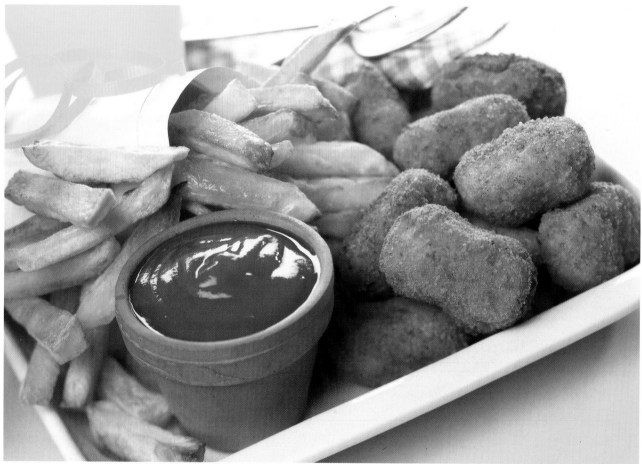

## oven fries

**6 medium potatoes (about 2¹/₂ lb)**
**¹/₄ cup olive oil**

Cut each potato lengthwise in ³/₈-inch-wide slices; cut slices into ³/₈-inch strips. Boil, steam or microwave strips until just tender; drain on paper towels.

Combine strips and oil in single layer on baking sheet; bake at 500°F about 45 minutes or until crisp and brown.

MAKES 12 SERVINGS

*Best made just before serving*

## chicken nuggets

**1 slice white bread**
**6 oz boneless chicken breast half, chopped**
**¹/₄ cup finely grated cheese**
**1 egg yolk**
**1 small potato, grated**
**1 small onion, grated**
**1 teaspoon poultry seasoning**
**1 teaspoon garlic salt**
**3 tablespoons packaged breadcrumbs**
**oil, for deep frying**

Cut crust from bread, chop coarsely. Blend or process bread, chicken and cheese until combined; transfer to medium bowl. Add egg, potato, onion and salt. Shape rounded tablespoons of mixture into nuggets; roll in breadcrumbs.

Deep fry nuggets, in batches, until chicken is cooked through and golden brown; drain on paper towels.

MAKES 16

Storage  Covered, in refrigerator, up to 2 days
Freeze  Uncooked nuggets suitable

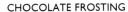
EGGLESS CHOCOLATE CAKE

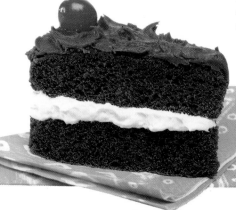

## funny faces

Using a 3¹/₂-inch cutter, cut rounds from slices of bread. "Draw" food faces using the following toppings.

CARROT TOP  grated carrot, green onion, tomato, parsley, cheese slice, cream cheese and poultry seasoning
LITTLE BOY  cheese slice, tomato, and Vegemite (see Glossary)
KITTY CAT  peanut butter, sliced banana, lemon rind and raspberry jam
GRIZZLY BEAR  chocolate hazelnut spread, white chocolate patties and red and white jelly beans

## eggless chocolate cake

*This cake is best eaten on the day it is made.*

**2 cups self-rising flour**
**¹/₄ cup cocoa**
**¹/₂ cup superfine sugar**
**1 ¹/₄ cups boiling water**
**3 tablespoons golden syrup or honey**
**1 teaspoon baking soda**
**¹/₃ cup butter, melted**
**1 teaspoon vanilla extract**
**¹/₂ cup cream, whipped**

CHOCOLATE FROSTING
**3 tablespoons finely chopped dark chocolate**
**2 tablespoons butter**
**³/₄ cup powdered sugar**
**1¹/₂ tablespoons cocoa**
**1¹/₂ tablespoons milk**
**¹/₂ teaspoon vanilla extract**

Grease two 8-inch round layer cake pans, line bottoms with parchment paper. Sift flour, cocoa and sugar into medium bowl; whisk in combined water, syrup, baking soda, butter and vanilla.

Divide mixture between prepared pans; bake, uncovered, at 325°F 25 minutes. Let cakes stand 10 minutes; turn onto wire rack to cool. Layer cooled cakes with whipped cream; top with Chocolate Frosting.

**Chocolate Frosting**  Combine chocolate and butter in small pan; stir over low heat until chocolate is melted. Sift sugar and cocoa into small bowl; stir in chocolate mixture, milk and vanilla. Cover, refrigerate 15 minutes or until frosting thickens.

**Freeze**  Unfrosted cakes suitable

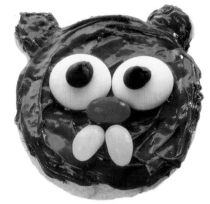
GRIZZLY BEAR

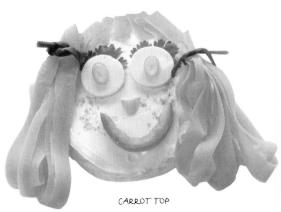
CARROT TOP

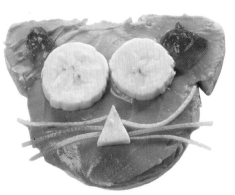
PUSSY CAT

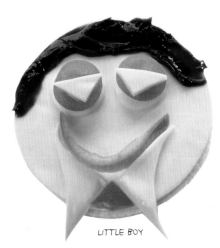
LITTLE BOY

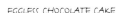

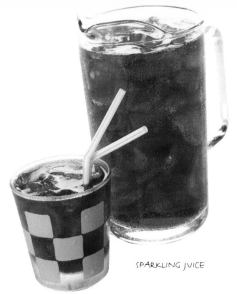

SPARKLING JUICE

## sparkling juice

Pour equal parts of apple-black currant or grape juice with soda or mineral water in a large pitcher; chill with ice cubes.

## candied popcorn

**3 tablespoons vegetable oil**
**1/2 cup popcorn**
**2 cups superfine sugar**
**1 cup water**
**1/2 teaspoon food coloring**

Heat oil in large pan; pop popcorn, covered, shaking pan occasionally, until popping stops. Transfer to large bowl. Combine sugar, water and food coloring in medium heavy-bottomed pan; stir over heat, without boiling, until sugar is dissolved. Bring to boil; boil, uncovered, about 15 minutes or until temperature reaches 325°F on candy thermometer (a teaspoon of mixture will crack when dropped into a cup of cold water). Allow bubbles to subside; add popcorn, stirring to coat with toffee mixture. When popcorn mixture has crystalized and separated, spread on foil-lined baking sheet.

MAKES 6 CUPS

**Storage** Airtight container up to 3 days

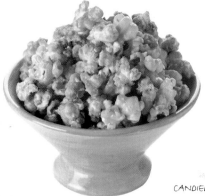

CANDIED POPCORN

## wieners

Place cocktail wieners in pan, cover with cold water; cook, uncovered, until water is just below boiling point, drain. Cut wieners into small pieces for very young children. A cute way to serve wieners to older children is to insert a popsicle stick into each cocktail wiener; serve with catsup for dipping.

Alternatively, serve mini hot dogs. Slice hot dog rolls lengthwise almost through; cut crosswise into thirds. Place one cocktail wiener in each piece; top with catsup and grated cheese.

WIENERS

SESAME CHICKEN MEATBALLS

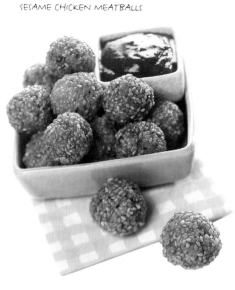

## monkey tails

**5 small firm bananas,**
**halved crosswise**
**7 oz milk chocolate patties**
**3 tablespoons vegetable oil**
**nonpareils, to decorate**
**colored sprinkles, to decorate**

Insert a popsicle stick into the bottom of each banana half. Melt chocolate in medium bowl over pan of simmering water; stir in oil. Dip bananas in chocolate mixture, one at a time, using a spoon to coat evenly. Decorate with nonpareils and sprinkles, as desired. Place on baking sheet; cover, refrigerate until set.

MAKES 10

## sesame chicken meatballs

**6 oz boneless chicken breast**
**half, chopped**
**1/2 teaspoon fish sauce**
**1/2 teaspoon sweet chili sauce**
**1 teaspoon lime juice**
**1 clove garlic, crushed**
**1 1/2 tablespoons shredded**
**fresh basil**
**3 tablespoons sesame seeds**
**vegetable oil, for deep frying**

Blend or process chicken, sauce, juice, garlic and basil until almost smooth. Using hands, roll rounded teaspoons of chicken mixture into ball; roll ball in sesame seeds. Place on baking sheet; repeat process with remaining mixture.
Deep-fry chicken meatballs, in batches, until cooked through and browned lightly; drain on paper towels.

MAKES 18

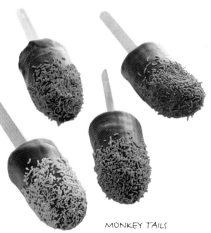

MONKEY TAILS

# the party package

The type of party that you hold will naturally vary according to the age of the child, so when planning your party, always bear in mind the age of the guest of honor and what he or she is able to do.

As a general rule, toddlers do not need elaborate parties and although the accompanying adults might appreciate your hours of culinary efforts, the little ones will not. They tend to handle everything, take one or two bites and make an almighty mess – disheartening to the cook and entirely predictable!

Since parties are sociable occasions, by all means provide a snack for the adults, but keep the food for the 2-year-olds very simple and try not to provide too much sugar. Excited toddlers can become very wound up after a sugary party – definite candidates for tears before bedtime!

Parties for 3- to 5-year-olds really start to be fun, as the children excitedly anticipate the occasion and enjoy the idea of fancy dress and other theme parties. Involve the birthday child in the preparations as much as possible, such as designing an invitation that can then be photocopied and distributed, or helping to decorate hats or fillling party bags. Enlist their opinion on the cake and party food as well, but remember that excitement will still rule the day and a great deal will not be eaten. Do not be too ambitious.

Food that is easy to handle and not too fussy is the sensible way to go, with a mix of both salty and sweet things. Children also love to take a party bag home with them. This does not have to be another sugar hit – small, inexpensive toys and novelty items will be just as popular.

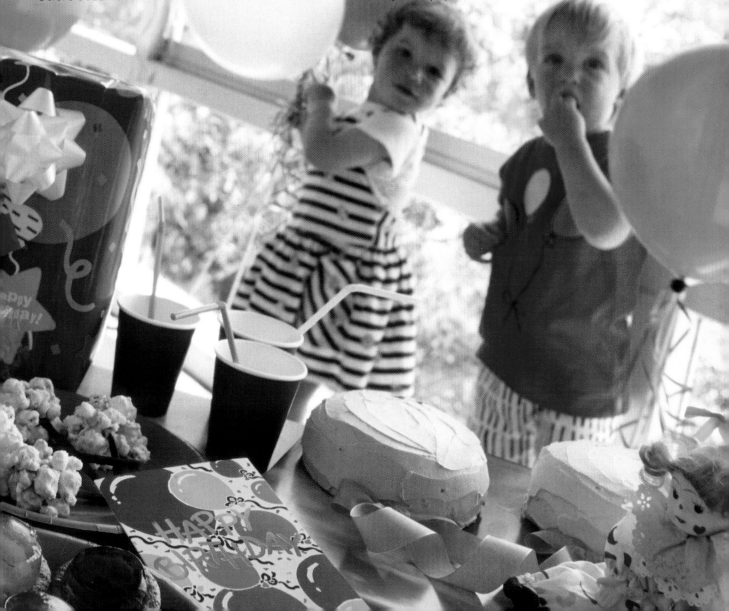

## little green frogs

*You need the ingredients listed on the packet
of cake mix for this recipe.*

**1 lb package Chocolate Cake
mix**
**3/4 cup butter**
**2 1/4 cups powdered
sugar**
**3 tablespoons milk**
**green food coloring**
**white marshmallows**
**chocolate chips**
**M & M's**

Line two 12-cup (1/3-cup capacity)
cupcake tins with cupcake liners. Make
cake according to directions on package;
divide mixture among cupcake liners.
Bake at 350°F 25 minutes; turn cupcakes
onto wire rack to cool.

Meanwhile, beat softened butter in
medium bowl with electric mixer until
smooth and pale. With motor running,
gradually beat in powdered sugar and
milk; tint with food coloring.

Top cupcakes with frosting. Using a
small knife, cut out a mouth shape from
each cupcake. Decorate with chocolate
chips, marshmallows and M & M's.

MAKES 24

**Storage** Airtight container up to 3 days
**Freeze** Unfrosted cupcakes suitable

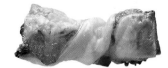

CHEESE TWISTS

## cheese twists

**1 sheet unfrozen, prepackaged
puff pastry**
**1 1/2 tablespoons catsup**
**1/2 cup coarsely grated
cheddar cheese**
**2 teaspoons milk**

Cut pastry in half. Spread one half with
catsup; sprinkle with cheese. Top with
remaining pastry; press down firmly.

Cut pastry into 12 strips; cut each
strip in half. Twist strips then place, 3/4
inch apart, on lightly greased baking
sheets; brush with milk. Bake,
uncovered, at 450°F about 10
minutes or until browned lightly.
Serve warm or at room temperature.

MAKES 24

**Storage** Airtight container up to 2 days
**Freeze** Unbaked twists suitable

## cassata cones

**1/2 gallon Neapolitan ice cream**
**1/4 cup green glace cherries,
chopped**
**1/4 cup red glace cherries,
chopped**
**1/4 cup dark chocolate chips,
chopped**
**12 small ice cream cones**
**1/4 cup dark chocolate-flavored
ice cream topping**
**1/4 cup white chocolate-flavored
ice cream topping**

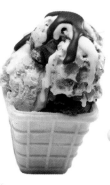

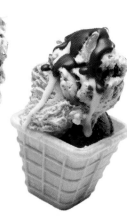

CASSATA CONES

Place vanilla third of Neapolitan ice
cream in medium bowl. Using a slotted
spoon, press down on ice cream until
just soft; add cherries and chocolate
chips, stir until combined. Return ice
cream, covered, to freezer until
set. Just before serving,
place 2 tablespoons of
chocolate ice cream in
bottom of each
cone. Next, place
2 tablespoons of
strawberry on
top of the
chocolate,
then top with
2 tablespoons
of vanilla ice
cream mixture. Drizzle
each cone with, first, dark
chocolate then white chocolate ice
cream topping; serve immediately.

MAKES 12

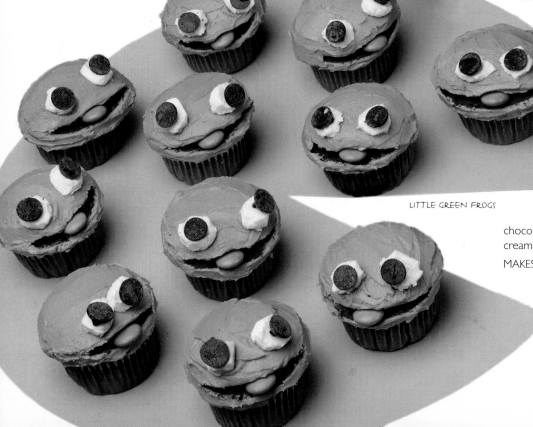

LITTLE GREEN FROGS

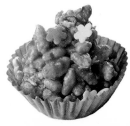

## chocolate rice crispy treats

**1 cup rice crispies**
**1/3 cup powdered sugar**
**1/4 cup dried coconut**
**2 teaspoons cocoa**
**1/4 cup vegetable shortening**
**sugar snowflakes, to decorate**

Combine rice crispies, sugar, coconut and cocoa in a large bowl. Heat shortening in small pan, uncovered, over low heat until melted; stir into dry ingredients, mix well. Spoon mixture into small paper tartlet liners; decorate with snowflakes. Refrigerate until set.

MAKES 18

**Storage** Airtight container, in refrigerator, up to 1 week

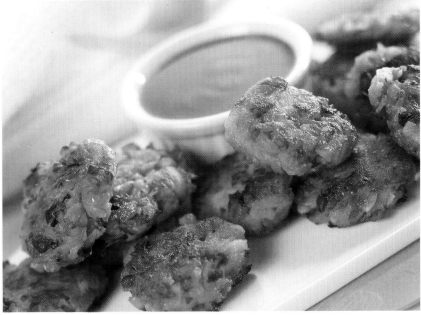

VEGETABLE PATTIES

## vegetable patties

**1 tablespoon butter**
**2 green onions, sliced thinly**
**1/2 cup coarsely grated orange sweet potato**
**1/2 cup coarsely grated potato**
**3 tablespoons finely chopped toasted pine nuts**
**1 egg yolk**
**3 tablespoons all-purpose flour**
**3 tablespoons vegetable oil**

Heat butter in medium pan; cook onion, sweet potato, potato and nuts, stirring, about 5 minutes or until potato is tender, cool. Stir in egg yolk and flour. Using floured hand, shape rounded teaspoons of mixture into balls; flatten slightly.

Heat oil in medium pan; fry patties, in batches, until browned both sides and cooked through. Drain on paper towels; serve with plum or sweet and sour sauce, if desired.

MAKES 20

**Storage** Covered, in refrigerator, up to 2 days

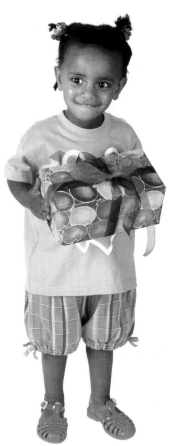

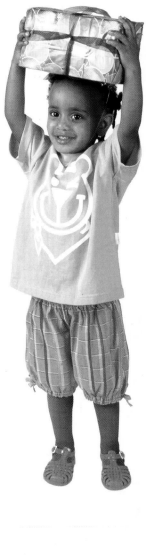

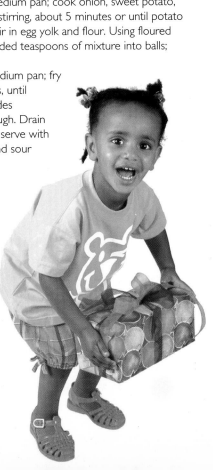

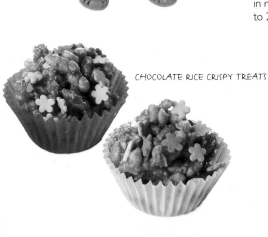

CHOCOLATE RICE CRISPY TREATS

## orange sorbet cups

**4 medium oranges, halved**
**1/3 cup cold water**
**3/4 cup superfine sugar**
**1/4 cup light corn syrup**
**1 cup warm water**
**2 egg whites, beaten lightly**

Squeeze oranges, reserving the halves; strain and reserve juice (you need 2 cups orange juice for this recipe). Scoop out and discard any remaining pulp from orange halves; reserve skin halves. Combine the cold water, sugar and syrup in small pan; heat, stirring, without boiling, until sugar dissolves. Simmer, uncovered, without stirring, 4 minutes. Stir in the warm water then the reserved juice. Pour mixture into shallow metal pan, cover with foil; freeze until just set. Working quickly, blend or process mixture with egg whites until smooth; scoop into orange skins, place on tray, return to freezer until set.

MAKES 8

## milk fruit log

**1/3 cup finely chopped dried apricots**
**1/4 cup finely chopped pitted dates**
**1/2 cup raisins, chopped finely**
**2 teaspoons finely chopped red glace cherries**
**3 tablespoons boiling water**
**1/4 cup skim milk powder**
**1/2 cup dried coconut**
**1 teaspoon vanilla extract**
**1/2 cup dried coconut, extra**

Combine apricots, dates, raisins and cherries in a medium mixing bowl. Pour the water into bowl, mix well; let stand 10 minutes. Stir in milk powder, coconut and vanilla. Roll rounded teaspoons of mixture into balls; dip into extra coconut. Refrigerate until firm.

MAKES 25

**Storage** Airtight container, in refrigerator, up to 1 week

☺ TIP Scissors make chopping dried fruit a breeze.

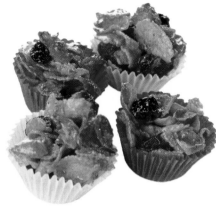

GOLDEN RAISIN CRUNCHIES

## golden raisin crunchies

**1 tablespoon butter**
**1 1/2 tablespoons honey**
**1 1/2 tablespoons brown sugar**
**1 cup corn flakes**
**1/4 cup golden raisins**

Place 18 small paper cupcake liners on baking sheet. Combine butter, honey and sugar in small pan; stir over heat until butter is melted. Add corn flakes and golden raisins; mix gently, spoon mixture into cupcake liners. Bake, uncovered, at 350°F about 10 minutes or until browned lightly.

MAKES 18

**Storage** Airtight container up to 1 week

## rocky road

**1/2 cup dried coconut**
**7 oz small multi-colored marshmallows**
**1/2 cup mixed glace cherries, chopped finely**
**1/4 cup unsalted roasted peanuts, chopped finely**
**13 oz milk chocolate, melted**

Grease 9" x 12" cake pan, cover bottom with parchment paper. Combine coconut, marshmallows, cherries and peanuts in large bowl. Stir in chocolate; spread mixture into prepared pan. Cover; refrigerate 30 minutes or until set. Break into small pieces to serve.

**Storage** Airtight container, in refrigerator, up to 1 week

**Delete nuts if serving to children under 5 years of age**

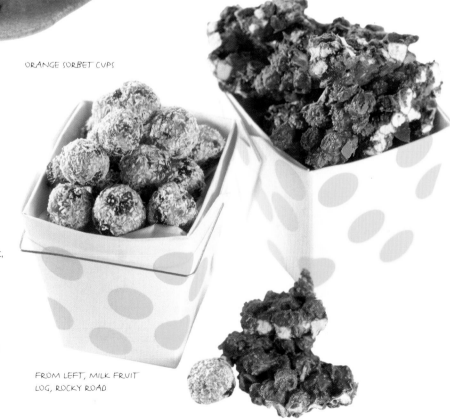

ORANGE SORBET CUPS

FROM LEFT, MILK FRUIT LOG, ROCKY ROAD

# one seagull

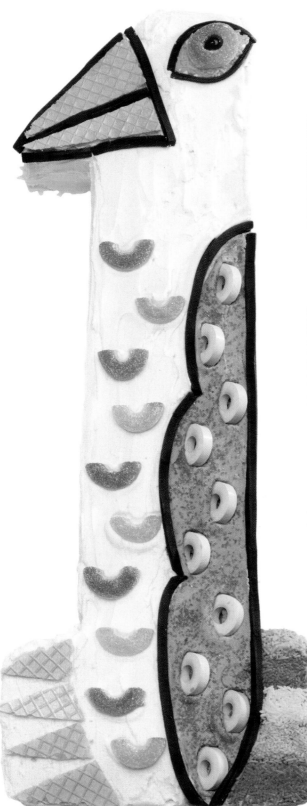

**FOR THE CAKE:**

**1 lb package Butter Cake mix**
**10" x 16" prepared board**
**1 batch Frosting (see page 113)**
**royal blue food coloring**

**TO DECORATE, YOU WILL NEED:**

**blue sugar crystals**
**4 wafer cookies**
**6 small orange and yellow gummi peach-o rings**
**1 roll spearmint Life Savers**
**pink, orange and yellow colored sprinkles**
**green decorating gel**
**1 black licorice twist**

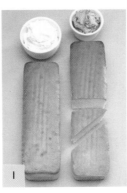

1

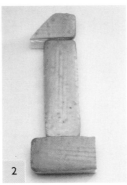

2

Grease two 3" x 10" loaf pans, line bottoms with parchment paper. Prepare cake according to directions on package; divide mixture evenly between prepared pans. Bake at 350°F about 35 minutes. Let cakes stand in pans 5 minutes; turn onto wire racks to cool.

Leave one cake whole, cut the other into 3 pieces, as shown, in diagram 1. Assemble cake on board, as shown in diagram 2, to form the figure 1.

Reserve 3/4 frosting; tint remaining frosting blue. Spread bird's wing with blue and remainder of bird with white frosting. Sprinkle wing with blue sugar crystals. Cut wafers into triangles to form bird's beak and feet. Reserve one gummi peach-o ring for eye; cut remaining rings in half. Push Life Savers halfway into wing and decorate body with gummi peach-o rings to resemble feathers.

Sprinkle pink, orange and yellow sprinkles in stripes along tail. Cut licorice twist into thin strips. Outline wing and beak with licorice. Use licorice to make shape of the eye, fill in with orange sprinkles; place gummi peach-o ring in position; fill in hole with green decorating gel.

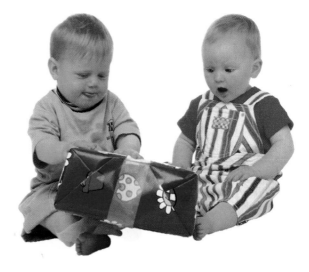

# Taller at two!

**FOR THE CAKE:**
**2 x 1 lb packages Butter Cake mix**
**14" x 18" prepared board**
**2 batches Frosting (see page 113)**
**orange food coloring**
**1/4 cup cocoa**

TO DECORATE, YOU WILL NEED:
**1 black licorice twist**
**1 white marshmallow**
**1 green nonpareil-covered gum drop**
**blue decorating gel**
**2 spearmint leaves**
**2 small bread sticks**
**2 small marshmallows**
**2 oz dark chocolate, melted**
**yellow sugar crystals**

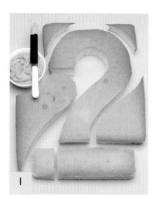

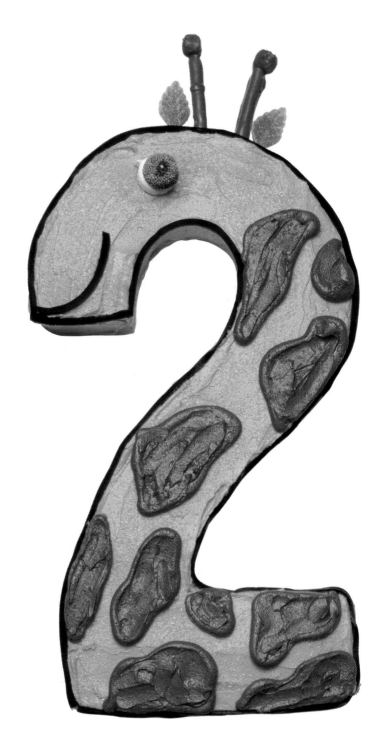

Grease 9" x 12" cake pan and 3" x 10" loaf pan, line bottoms with parchment paper. Using both packages, prepare cakes according to directions on package; pour into prepared pans. Bake at 350°F about 25 minutes for loaf pan and 40 minutes for cake pan. Let cakes stand in pans 5 minutes, turn onto wire racks to cool.

Cut out the figure 2 as shown above. Place cakes on prepared board.

Tint 3/4 of frosting with orange coloring; tint remaining frosting by stirring in sifted cocoa.

Spread top and side of cake with orange frosting. Spoon chocolate frosting into piping bag fitted with a small plain tip; pipe spots onto cake. Cut licorice twist into thin strips. Position strips to outline cake and make mouth.

Cut marshmallow in half, discard one half; place nonpareil-covered gum drop on top of remaining half. Pipe dot with blue gel on berry to complete eye; position on head. Insert toothpicks into bottom of spearmint leaves, position on head. Spear a small marshmallow on the end of each bread stick, then dip both in chocolate; place on parchment-lined baking sheet; let stand until chocolate is set. Position bread stick next to mint leaves to resemble horns. Sprinkle sugar crystals on orange frosting.

# Fishes for three

**FOR THE CAKE:**

**2 x 1 lb packages Butter Cake mix**
**10" x 16" prepared board**
**2 batches Frosting (see page 113)**
**royal blue food coloring**

**TO DECORATE, YOU WILL NEED:**

**4 peppermint Mentos**
**red decorating gel**
**4 apricot Roll-Ups**
**36 blue M & M's**
**5 ice cream wafers**
**1¹/₂ tablespoons orange coloured sprinkles**
**1 black licorice twist**
**2 teaspoons blue sugar crystals**

Grease two 8-inch ring cake pans, line bottoms with parchment paper. Using both packages, make cakes according to directions on package; divide evenly between pans. Bake at 350°F about 45 minutes.

Let cakes stand in pans 5 minutes, turn onto wire racks to cool. Cut out pieces and join as shown below to form the figure 3. Place cakes on prepared board. Tint ²/₃ frosting dark blue with food coloring; tint the remaining frosting a pale blue.

Spread cake with frosting as shown, reserve about 3 tablespoons of dark blue frosting. Place 2 mints on light blue frosting as eyes. Using red decorating gel, make large pupils on mints.

Cut two Roll-Ups into 4 fin-shaped pieces. Join 2 fins together with a little water. Place fins at the start of the dark blue icing on each end.

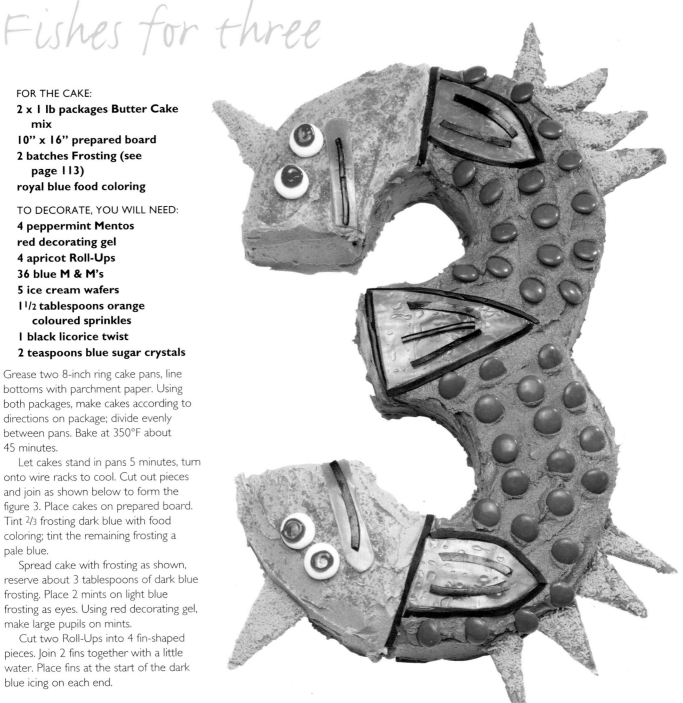

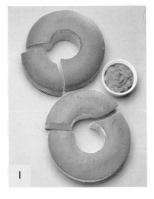

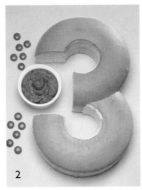

Cut two 2" x 3¹/₂" triangles from Roll-Ups. Join triangles together with a little water. Place on cake at the center of the figure 3 to resemble a tail.

Cut four ³/₈" x 2¹/₂" strips from remaining Roll-Ups, shape one end into a curve; join two pieces with a little water. Place Roll-Ups on each end to resemble a mouth. Place M & M's on cake to resemble scales. Cut wafers in half diagonally.

Place 8 pieces of wafer on top and bottom outer edge of cake, as shown, to form spines. Place 2 remaining wafer pieces on side of cake above eyes. Spread wafers with reserved frosting. Sprinkle wafer spines with orange sprinkles.

Cut licorice into thin pieces. Outline fins, tail and join of frostings; define fins, tail and mouth with licorice pieces. Sprinkle pale blue heads with blue sugar crystals.

# Tiger turns four

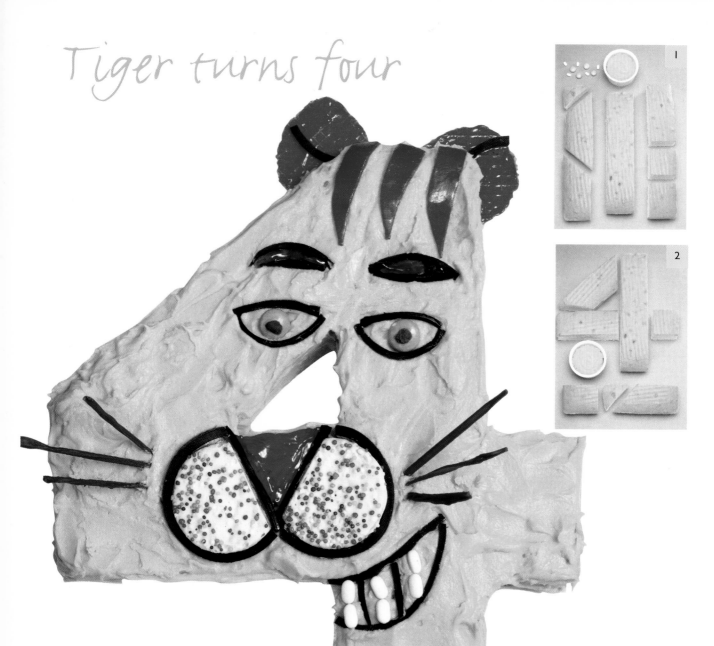

**FOR THE CAKE:**

**1 lb package Butter Cake mix**
**12" x 16" prepared board**
**2 batches frosting (see page 113)**
**yellow food coloring**

**TO DECORATE, YOU WILL NEED:**

**1 black licorice twist**
**green decorating gel**
**M & M's or Skittles**
**2 x 2-inch frosted cookies**
**4 pieces spaghetti**
**3 1/2 oz milk chocolate**
**red decorating gel**
**6 peppermint Tic Tacs**
**6-inch strip red Roll-Up**
**2 vanilla ice cream wafers**

Grease 8" x 12" cake pan, line the bottom with parchment paper. Prepare cake mix according to directions on package; pour into prepared pan. Bake at 350°F about 25 minutes. Let cake stand in pan 5 minutes; turn onto wire rack to cool.

Cut cake into 3 equal pieces lengthwise. Cut 2 pieces into 3 sections each, as shown in diagram 1. Assemble pieces on prepared board to make the figure 4, as shown in diagram 2. Tint frosting with yellow food coloring. Spread frosting over top and side of cake, fluff frosting with a fork to resemble fur.

Cut licorice twist into thin strips; position strips to outline eyebrows, eyes and mouth. Pipe green gel to complete eyebrows. Place M & M's or Skittles on cake to form eyes; dot with green gel to complete.

Cut a slice off each cookie, discard smaller piece; place larger cookie shapes on cake to form muzzle, outline with licorice. Make whiskers by breaking spaghetti pieces in half; roll in melted chocolate to coat, place on parchment, allow to set. Place spaghetti whiskers in position; spread red gel over nose to complete, use Tic Tacs to form teeth.

Cut fruit Roll-Up into 3 triangles; position on head to form stripes.

Cut each wafer into 1 1/2-inch circle. Pipe red gel over wafers, press into top of cake, place licorice stick on each ear to complete.

**FOR THE CAKE:**

**1 lb package Butter Cake mix**
**10" x 14" prepared board**
**2 batches Frosting (see below)**
**pink, green, black, blue and**
   **orange food colorings**

TO DECORATE, YOU WILL NEED:
**thin red licorice rope**
**1 black licorice twist**
**peppermint Tic Tacs**
**2 peppermint Mentos**
**blue decorating gel**
**2 small yellow banana Runts**
**2 nonpareil-covered gum drops**

Grease 8" ring cake pan and 3" x 10" loaf pan, line bottoms with parchment paper. Using both packages, prepare cake mix according to directions on package, divide mixture between pans. Bake at 350°F about 25 minutes. Stand cake in pans 5 minutes, turn onto wire racks to cool.

Cut out cake to form the figure 5 as shown in diagram 1. Assemble pieces on prepared board, as shown in diagram 2. Tint 1/2 frosting with pink coloring, 1/4 with green coloring, and a 1/4 cup of remaining frosting with black coloring. Of remaining frosting, tint 1/3 with blue coloring and remaining frosting with orange coloring.

Spread top and outer side of round cake with pink frosting. With remaining green frosting, make a 3/4" border on inside edge of round cake, and on top of cake to form mouth. Spread loaf cake top and sides with orange frosting and eye area with black frosting. Spoon remaining green frosting into piping bag fitted with a small plain tip; pipe below black for nose.

Spoon blue frosting into clean piping bag fitted with a small plain tip, pipe 6 lines dividing pink and orange frostings. Cut black licorice twist into thin strips. Position red licorice rope to outline mouth and black licorice strips to outline eyes.

*Gotcha! at five*

Cut remaining black licorice strips into small pieces to make whiskers. Arrange Tic Tacs to form teeth. Dot Mentos with blue gel to form eyes; place bananas above eyes for eyebrows and nonpareil-covered gum drops for ears.

**FROSTING**
**1/2 cup soft butter**
**1 1/2 cups powdered sugar**
**3 tablespoons milk**

Beat butter in small bowl with electric mixer until light in color; gradually beat in half the sugar, then the milk, then the remaining sugar. Flavor and color frosting as desired.

**Preparing cake boards** To make a cake easy to handle as well as more attractive, place it on a board which has been covered in decorative paper. We have given approximate cake board size with each recipe. Using Masonite or a similarly strong board, cut your paper 2 to 4 inches larger than the shaped board.

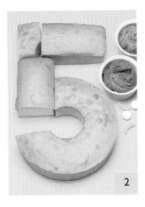

# glossary

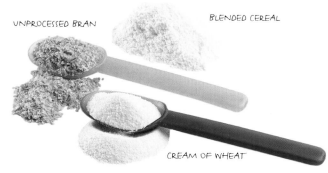

UNPROCESSED BRAN
BLENDED CEREAL
CREAM OF WHEAT

**APPLE-BLACK CURRANT JUICE**
a sweetened drink made from these two fruits, sweetener and water, with vitamin supplements.

**ANCHOVY PASTE** a paste made from fish, wheat flour, salt, flavour and coloring. Also known as fish paste.

**BANANA CHILI** a mild yellow/green banana-shaped chili. Also known as sweet banana peppers. Seeds and membranes should be discarded before use.

**BEANS, CANNED MIXED** a canned mix of red kidney, garbanzo, baby lima and butter beans.

**BEAN SPROUTS** also known as bean shoots; tender new growths of assorted beans and seeds germinated for consumption as sprouts. The most readily available are mung bean, soy bean, alfalfa and snow pea sprouts.

**BEEF**

**Blade steak** from the shoulder blade area; also chuck steak or roast.

**Corned** beef cut from the brisket or silverside cured in a piquantly flavored brine.

**Rib-eye steak** eye of the rib roast, sliced; also called spencer steak.

**BLANCHING** to partially cook food (usually vegetables and fruits) very briefly, in boiling water; then draining and plunging into cold water.

**BREADCRUMBS**

**Fresh** 1- or 2-day-old bread made into crumbs by grating or blending

**Packaged** fine-textured, crunchy, purchased, white breadcrumbs.

**BROWN-AND-SERVE ROLLS** commercially baked bread rolls that have been cooked to 80% of total cooking time.

**BUTTER** use salted or unsalted ("sweet") butter; 1 stick butter equals 1/2 cup or 4 ounces.

**CEREALS**

**Blended cereal** recommended first food for babies from 4 months. A dry mixture of ground rice, cornflour, soy flour, various vitamins and minerals.

**Bran flakes** a breakfast cereal based on processed wheat bran enriched with vitamins.

DARK CHOCOLATE

DARK CHOCOLATE CHIPS

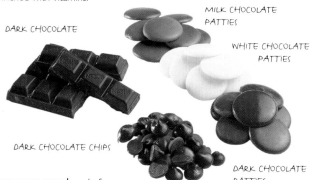

MILK CHOCOLATE PATTIES

WHITE CHOCOLATE PATTIES

DARK CHOCOLATE PATTIES

**Bran, unprocessed** made from the outer layer of a cereal, most often the husks of wheat, rice or oats.

**Corn flakes** breakfast cereal made from toasted corn.

Cream of wheat made from durum wheat milled into various textured granules, all of these finer than flour. Used to make couscous, good pastas, some kinds of gnocchi and many Middle-Eastern and Indian sweets

**Muesli/granola** breakfast cereal made from a mixture of raw or toasted grains, dried fruit, nuts, coconut and sugar.

**Rice crispies** breakfast cereal made from puffed rice, sugar, salt and malt extract, plus added vitamins and minerals.

**Rolled oats/oatmeal** whole oats grains steamed, rolled and flattened; used for making oatmeal mush or in baking.

**Shredded wheat** breakfast biscuits made from whole wheat, salt, sugar, malt extract and various vitamins and minerals.

**CHOCOLATE**

**Chocolate chips** also known as Choc Bits and chocolate morsels; available in milk, white and dark chocolate. Made of cocoa liquor, cocoa butter, sugar and an emulsifier, these hold their shape in baking and are ideal when used for decorating.

Cocoa cocoa powder.

Dark eating-quality chocolate; made of cocoa liquor, cocoa butter and sugar.

Patties available in milk, white and dark chocolate. Made of sugar, vegetable fats, milk solids, cocoa powder, butter oil and emulsifiers, these are good for melting and molding.

**CINNAMON SUGAR** combination of superfine sugar and ground cinnamon.

**COCONUT**

**Cream** available in cans and cartons; made from coconut and water.

**Dried** unsweetened, concentrated, dried and shredded coconut.

**Milk** pure, unsweetened coconut milk available in cans and cartons.

**COLESLAW DRESSING** commercially prepared mayonnaise-style dressing commonly used in cabbage and some fruit salads. Contains oil, sugar, vinegar, egg yolk, salt, cornflour, spices and skim milk powder.

**CORN STARCH** powdered starch from corn; used as a thickening agent in cooking.

**CORN SYRUP** a thick sweet syrup available in light or dark color, either can be substituted for the other; glucose syrup (liquid glucose) can be substituted.

**COUSCOUS** a fine, grain-like cereal product originating in North Africa; made from semolina rolled into balls.

**CRACKER BREAD** lavash; flat unleavened bread of Mediterranean origin.

SHREDDED WHEAT

CORN FLAKES

ROLLED OATS

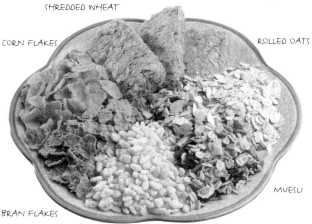

BRAN FLAKES

RICE CRISPIES

MUESLI

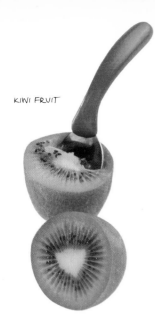

KIWI FRUIT

## CREAM

**Fresh** also known as pouring cream; has no additives like commercially thickened cream.

**Sour** a thick, commercially-cultured soured cream good for dips, toppings and baked cheesecakes.

**Thickened** a whipping cream containing a thickener.

**CURRY POWDER** a blend of ground, powdered spices used for convenience when making Indian food. Can consist of some or all of the following spices in varying proportions: dried chili, cinnamon, coriander, cumin, fennel, fenugreek, mace, cardamom and turmeric.

**EXTRACTS** also known as essences; generally the byproduct of distillation of plants.

**FARFALLE** bow-tie pasta

**FILO PASTRY** also known as phyllo; tissue-thin pastry sheets purchased chilled or frozen that are easy to work with and very versatile, lending themselves to both sweet and salty dishes.

**FISH FILLETS** fish pieces that have been boned and skinned.

## FLOUR

**All-purpose** plain flour made from wheat.

**All-purpose wholewheat** flour made from whole wheat that has no baking powder added.

**Rice** a very fine flour, made from ground white rice.

**Self-rising** all-purpose flour sifted with baking powder in the proportion of 1 cup flour to 2 teaspoons baking powder.

**FOOD COLORINGS** available in liquid, powdered and concentrated paste forms.

**FRENCH ONION SOUP MIX** a packaged soup mix often added to meat and poultry dishes for flavor and as a thickening agent.

**GARBANZOS** also called chick peas, hummus or channa; an irregularly round, sandy-colored legume used extensively in Mediterranean, Hispanic and Indian cooking.

**GELATIN** we used powdered gelatin. It is also available in sheet form known as leaf gelatin.

**GHERKIN** sometimes known as a cornichon; young, dark-green, extremely tiny cucumbers grown especially for pickling.

**GNOCCHI** Italian "dumplings" made of potatoes, semolina or flour; can be cooked in boiling water or baked with a sauce.

**GOLDEN SYRUP** a byproduct of refined sugar cane; pure maple syrup, corn syrup or honey can be substituted.

## ICE MAGIC

**Chocolate** chocolate-flavored ice cream coating made of vegetable oils, sugar, cocoa, skim milk powder and emulsifiers.

**White** white chocolate-flavored ice cream coating made of vegetable fat, sugar, milk solids, lactose, emulsifiers and flavors.

**JELLO** fruit-flavored gelatin crystals available from supermarkets.

**KIWI FRUIT** furry, tan-colored fruit with sweet, tart green flesh; also known as Chinese gooseberry.

**LADYFINGERS** Italian-style sponge cake "fingers"; also known as Savoiardi or Savoy biscuits.

## LAMB

**Chop** small, tender rib cutlet.

**Diced** cubed lean meat.

**Forequarter chop** medium-sized chop cut from the shoulder.

**Rack** row of rib chops.

**Shank** forequarter leg.

**LENTILS, RED** a small dried red/orange legumes originating in the Middle East.

**MARMITE** see Vegemite.

**MEXICAN-STYLE CHILI POWDER** a blend of ground chilli, cumin, oregano and garlic. Used in cooking to impart a Mexican-like flavor to food.

## MILK

**Condensed** canned, milk of thick consistency which has been evaporated and sweetened.

**Formula** a formulated breast milk substitute sold in powdered form.

**Skim Milk Powder** we used dried milk powder having 1% fat content when dry and 0.1% when reconstituted.

**MIXED DRIED FRUIT** a combination of golden raisins, dark raisins, currants, mixed peel and cherries.

**MUFFIN, ENGLISH** a round, flat yeast cake, baked on both sides; often confused with the batter-based crumpet.

**NEAPOLITAN ICE CREAM** a widely available, commercially prepared, 3-flavor combination ice cream. Usually strawberry, vanilla and chocolate.

**NONPAREILS** tiny candy balls sprinkled on cakes and cookies for decoration.

## NOODLES

**Bean thread** also called cellophane; made from green mung bean flour. Good softened in soups and salads or deep-fried with vegetables.

**Instant** Also known as ramen, a crinkly or straight dried wheat noodle. Are referred to as 2-minute noodles in reference to their short cooking time.

**Rice noodle** also known as rice-flour or rice-stick noodles; made from ground rice. Sold dried, they are best either deep-fried or soaked then stir-fried or used in soups.

## OIL

**Extra virgin and virgin** the highest quality olive oils, obtained from the first pressings of the olives.

**Olive** mono-unsaturated; made from the pressing of tree-ripened olives. Especially good for everyday cooking and as an ingredient. Extra Light or Light describes the mild flavor, not the fat levels.

**Peanut** pressed from ground peanuts; most commonly used oil in Asian cooking because of its high smoke point.

**Sesame** also called Dark Sesame Oil; made from roasted, crushed, white sesame seeds; used as a flavoring rather than a cooking medium.

**Vegetable** any of a number of cooking oils having a plant rather than animal source.

## ONION

**Green** also known as scallion or (incorrectly) shallot; an immature onion picked before the bulb has fully formed, having a long, bright-green edible stalk.

**Red** also known as Spanish, red Spanish or Bermuda onion; a sweet-flavored, large, purple-red onion that is particularly good eaten raw in salads.

**Yellow** gold-skinned onion with a strong flavor.

**PINE NUT** also known as pignoli; small, cream-colored kernels obtained from the cones of different varieties of pine trees.

## PLAIN SWEET BISCUITS

uniced, plain, packaged biscuit, sometimes sprinkled with sugar.

**POLENTA** a flour-like cereal made of ground corn; similar to cornmeal but coarser and darker in color; also the name of the dish made from it.

**POPPADUMS** sun-dried wafers made from a combination of lentil and rice flours, oil and spices; can be deep-fried or "puffed" in the microwave oven.

**POPPING CORN** dried kernels of a particular strain of corn which pop when heated.

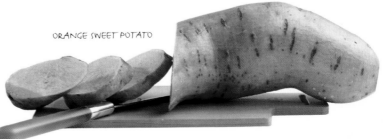

ORANGE SWEET POTATO

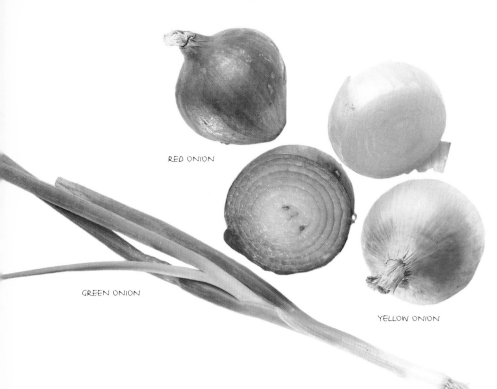

RED ONION

GREEN ONION

YELLOW ONION

**Superfine** very finely granulated table sugar.

**TAHINI** a rich, buttery paste made from crushed sesame seeds; used in making hummus and other Middle-Eastern sauces.

**TOMATO PASTE** triple-concentrated tomato puree used to flavor soups, stews, sauces and casseroles.

**TORTELLINI** small rounds of pasta, filled, sealed, then shaped into rounds.

**TORTILLA** thin, round unleavened bread originating in Mexico; some are made from wheat flour and others from corn.

**VEGEMITE** yeast extract spread made in Australia; found in specialty shops or upscale grocery stores; very salty; use sparingly; may be substituted with Marmite or Promite, similar products made in Great Britain.

**VEGETABLE SHORTENING** a fat made from vegetable oils, such as cottonseed or coconut oil, which is solid at room temperature.

## WIENERS

**Cocktail** a lightly smoked pre-cooked sausage made from a mixture of pork, beef or veal, starch, salt and various additives in red casing. Usually about 2–3 inches in length.

**Hot dog** a fine-textured smoked pre-cooked sausage made from a mixture of pork, beef and veal, selected spices, starch, salt and various additives in red casing. Usually about 6 inches in length.

## PORK

**Boneless chop** skinless, boneless eye-fillet cut from the loin.

**PROMITE** see Vegemite.

**RED CURRANT JELLY** a preserve made from red currants used as a glaze for desserts and meats or as a part of a sauce.

**RICE PAPER** mostly from Vietnam (banh trang). Made from a paste of ground rice and water and stamped into rounds, with a woven pattern. Dipped briefly in water, they become pliable wrappers for fried food and for eating fresh vegetables.

**SATAY MARINADE** commercially prepared thin version of the traditional mixture of peanuts, sugar, soy sauce, salt, garlic, chili, spices and vinegar.

## SAUCES

**Barbecue** spicy tomato-based sauce used to marinate, baste or as an accompaniment.

**Catsup** made from tomatoes, vinegar, sugar and spices.

**Fish** also called nam pla or nuoc nam; made from pulverized salted fermented fish, most often anchovies. Has a pungent smell and strong taste; use sparingly. There are many kinds, each of varying intensity.

**Hoisin** thick, sweet and spicy Chinese paste made from salted fermented soy beans, onions and garlic; used as a marinade or to baste, or to accent stir-fries and barbecued or roasted foods.

**Oyster** Asian in origin, this rich, brown sauce is made from oysters and their brine, cooked with salt and soy sauce, and thickened with starches.

**Plum** thick, sweet and sour dipping sauce made from plums, vinegar, sugar, chilies and spices.

**Soy** made from fermented soy beans. Several variations are available in most supermarkets and Asian food stores.

**Sweet chili** mild, Thai-type sauce made from red chilies, sugar, garlic and vinegar.

**Teriyaki** homemade or commercially bottled sauce usually made from soy sauce, corn syrup, vinegar, ginger and other spices; it imparts a distinctive glaze when brushed on grilled meats.

**Worcestershire** thin, dark-brown spicy sauce used as a seasoning for meat, gravies and cocktails and as a condiment.

**SCONES** also known as biscuits.

## SPRING ROLL WRAPPERS

are also sometimes called egg roll wrappers; they come in various sizes and can be purchased fresh or frozen from Asian supermarkets. Made from a delicate wheat-based pastry, they can be used for making gow gee, samosas and spring rolls.

**STOCK** 1 cup stock is the equivalent of 1 cup water plus 1 crumbled stock cube (or 1 teaspoon stock powder).

**SUGAR** we used coarse, granulated table sugar, also known as crystal sugar, unless otherwise specified.

**Brown** an extremely soft, fine granulated sugar retaining its molasses flavor.

**Powdered sugar** also known as confectioners' sugar; granulated sugar crushed together with a small amount (about 3%) cornflour added.

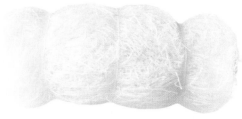

BEAN THREAD NOODLES

RICE NOODLES

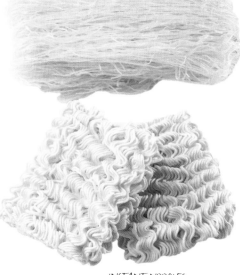

INSTANT NOODLES

# index

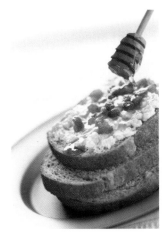

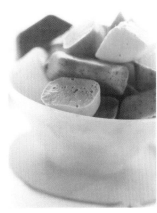

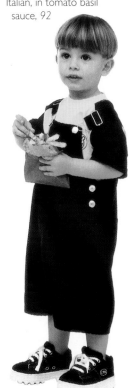

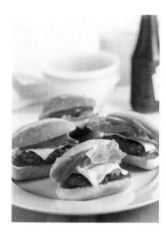

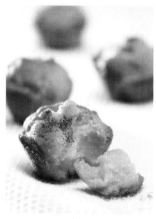

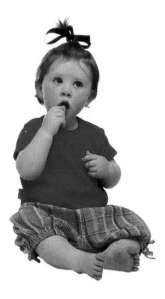

# Add these new Cole's Home Library mini menu cookbooks to your collection

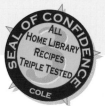

## mini books
## maxi results

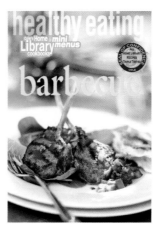

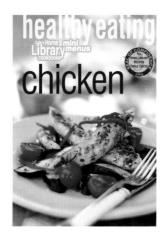

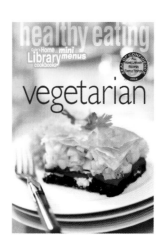

fit for life – **healthy eating**

**make it tonight** – good food fast

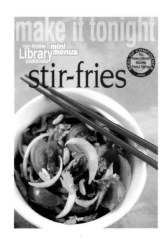

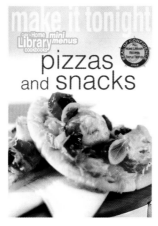

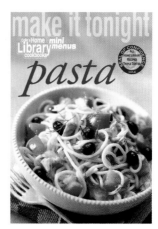

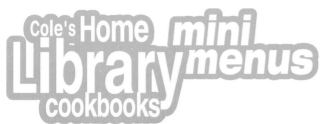

on sale at selected retailers and supermarkets

# More great new titles from

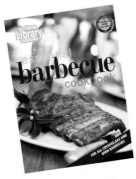

## COOKERY

### The Essential Barbecue Cookbook

Enjoying the best the barbecue has to offer, this innovative collection of recipes is all you need to prepare fabulous dishes and outdoor meals. *The Essential Barbecue Cookbook* covers cooking beef, veal, poultry, lamb, seafood, pork and vegetables, along with taste-tempting breads and desserts. All your questions are answered about gas and charcoal cooking fuel sources, grill gadgets and we show you how to buy and look after your grill. Barbecuing is no longer a summer-time-only pursuit. So, anytime of the year, fire up the barbecue and impress family and friends with these easy-to-prepare recipes for all open kettle and gas grills. Over 180 recipes, including full glossary and index.

ISBN 1-56426-153-0          $11.95

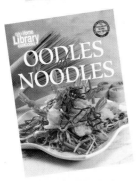

### Meals-in-Minutes

Fast, simple and healthy are the catch cries for today's busy lifestyle. *Meals-in-Minutes* is specially designed for the enthusiastic cook with little time. This exciting collection proves that fast food can also be good food – good for you, good to eat, good and tasty. Some of the recipes featured take just a few minutes while others can be prepared ahead of time for quick dining after work or when family meals are needed in a hurry. All recipes use simple ingredients for exciting results and have all been triple tested for flavor and easy preparation. *Meals-in Minutes* will become a kitchen standby. Over 180 recipes, including full glossary and index.

ISBN 1-56426-150-6-0          $11.95

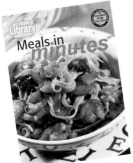

### Oodles of Noodles

Noodles are the new pasta! Versatile and delicious, there's an almost limitless variety of noodles available: fresh or dried, rice, wheat or flour, egg or eggless. With this Home Library original, you'll learn to use your noodles and your culinary success will be assured. This special collection covers soups, starters and finger food, salads, stir-fries and main meals all featuring fabulous noodles in all their guises. Meat dishes, chicken and other poultry, seafood and vegetarian delights are all included. Samples of each noodle, before and after cooking, make this collection particularly easy to use and we also include shopping and noodle preparation tips. Over 120 traditional and innovative recipes, including full glossary and index.

ISBN 1-56426-151-4          $11.95

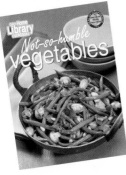

### Not-So-Humble Vegetables

This A-Z stroll through the vegie patch is both a visual and culinary treat. Starting at A for Artichoke through to Z for Zucchini, this special collection will tempt all the senses. Menu planning becomes very easy and exciting with this huge array of main dishes, accompaniments and side dishes. With new varieties readily available in most supermarkets and green grocers, enjoying the world of vegetables is becoming a favorite pastime of city dwellers and suburbanites alike. No longer second-best to meat and seafood, vegetables now step into the spotlight and their infinite variety of tastes, textures and colours is dazzling. Over 180 recipes, including glossary, nutrition guide and index.

ISBN 1-56426-152-2          $11.95

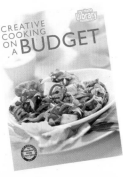

### Creative Cooking on a Budget

Cooking on a budget can have a fun and creative side. The challenge of feeding family and friends delicious and exciting meals without spending a fortune brings out the inventor as well as the chef in the most hesitant of cooks. These triple-tested healthy and achievable recipes are as affordable as they are delectable. They use readily available ingredients to make exciting and inexpensive meals, and you will be inspired to dream up your own creations. These fabulous recipes will also convince you that home cooking is not only infinitely better but far more inexpensive than over-priced take-out foods. Over 130 recipes, with hints on how to keep cooking costs low with no sacrifice of taste, full glossary and index.

ISBN 1-56426-157-3          $11.95